W9-CES-026

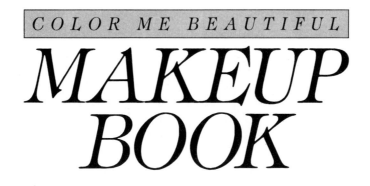

COLOR ME BEAUTIFUL

MAKEUP BOOK

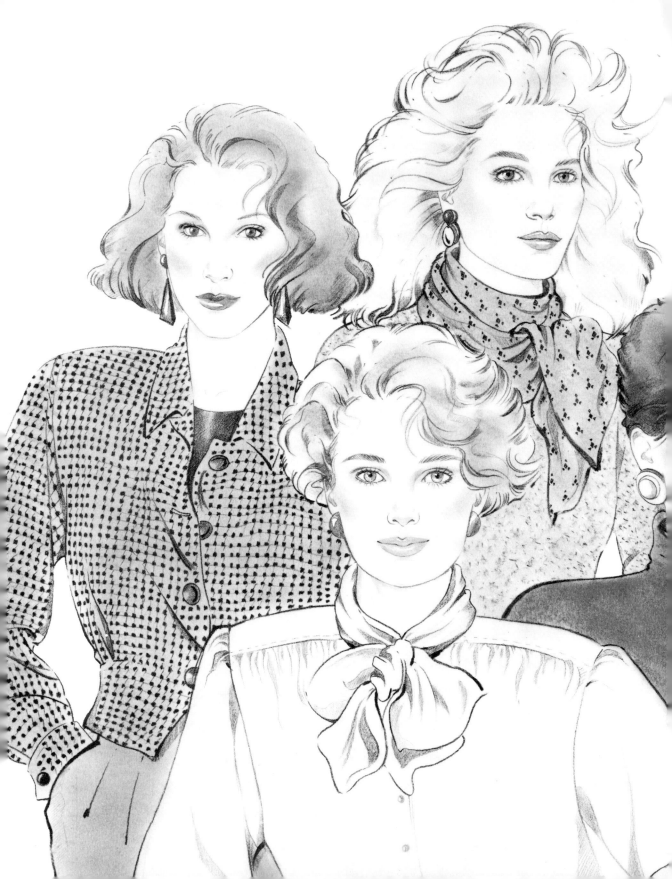

COLOR ME BEAUTIFUL

MAKEUP BOOK

CAROLE JACKSON

BALLANTINE BOOKS • NEW YORK

Sale of this book without a front cover may be unauthorized. If this book is coverless, it may have been reported to the publisher as "unsold or destroyed" and neither the author nor the publisher may have received payment for it.

Also by Carole Jackson

Color Me Beautiful
Color for Men

Photography by Michael Latil, Michael Latil Photography, Alexandria, Virginia.
Illustrations by Marika Hahn.
Thanks to Nancy DiAntonio and Barbara Murray for appearing in *The Color Me Beautiful Makeup Book*.

All other models are from The Artist Agency, Georgetown, D.C.:

Sheron George	Jill Reuther
Megan Bartsch	Doreen Totaro
Diane Lawlor	Jennifer Van Horn
Rebecca Peed	

Styling by Sharran Weber. Makeup by Barbara York. Hair design by Bob Starke and Sharran Weber.

Clothing courtesy of Inge's of Alexandria and Woodward & Lothrop, and Color Me Beautiful Apparel. Model's scarves by Color Me Beautiful, Europe.

Copyright © 1987 by Carole Jackson
Illustrations copyright © 1987 by Marika Hahn
Photography copyright © 1987 by Michael Latil Photography

All rights reserved under International and Pan-American Copyright Conventions. Published in the United States by Ballantine Books, a division of Random House, Inc., New York, and simultaneously in Canada by Random House of Canada Limited, Toronto.

COLOR ME BEAUTIFUL is a registered trademark of Color Me Beautiful, Inc.

Library of Congress Catalog Card Number: 87-91179

ISBN: 0-345-34842-7

Cover design by James R. Harris
Cover photo by Michael Latil
Text design by Michaelis/Carpelis Design Associates

Manufactured in the United States of America

First Edition: January 1988
10 9 8 7 6

This book is dedicated to my Color Me Beautiful
consultants worldwide, whose caring
attitudes and dedication to excellence have
given life to our company and enabled
us to carry out our mission.

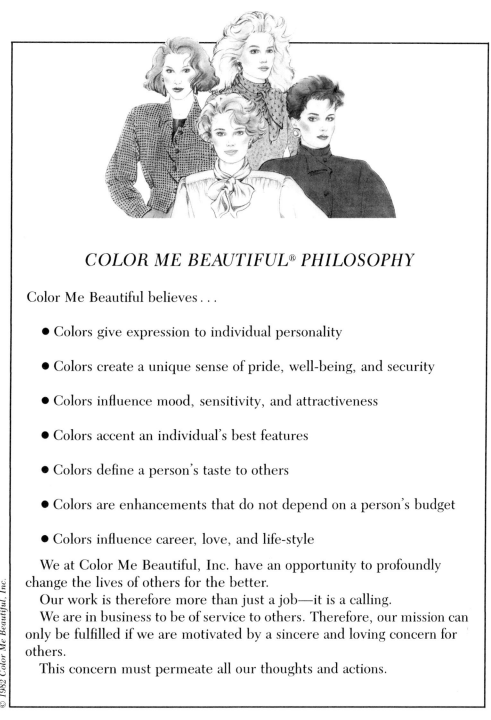

COLOR ME BEAUTIFUL® PHILOSOPHY

Color Me Beautiful believes . . .

- Colors give expression to individual personality

- Colors create a unique sense of pride, well-being, and security

- Colors influence mood, sensitivity, and attractiveness

- Colors accent an individual's best features

- Colors define a person's taste to others

- Colors are enhancements that do not depend on a person's budget

- Colors influence career, love, and life-style

We at Color Me Beautiful, Inc. have an opportunity to profoundly change the lives of others for the better.

Our work is therefore more than just a job—it is a calling.

We are in business to be of service to others. Therefore, our mission can only be fulfilled if we are motivated by a sincere and loving concern for others.

This concern must permeate all our thoughts and actions.

© 1982 Color Me Beautiful, Inc.

Acknowledgments

Getting a book from the word processor to the bookstore is always a team effort! I am indebted to the following people for their help in bringing the philosophy of Color Me Beautiful makeup to the printed page:

The people at Ballantine Books: Joëlle Delbourgo, Editor-in-Chief, who endures my artistic temperament with grace and charm; Fred Dodnick, Director of Production; Stephen McNabb, Managing Editor; Jimmy Harris, Art Director; and Karen Hwa, Editorial Assistant and most patient person.

For book design, Sylvain Michaelis and Irene Carpelis of Michaelis/Carpelis Design Associates; for their editing and enthusiasm, Nellie Sabin, Elisa Petrini, and Ravin Korothy; for research and writing, Sandy Fitzgerald, Nancy DiAntonio, and Andrea Lentz; for consulting on the hair chapter, Dennis Lucier of For Hair Only; and for typing and moral support, Liz Singley and Maggy Linka.

For editing, proofreading, and love, Jean Halliburton, my beautiful mother; for special friendship and leading Color Me Beautiful to greatness, Steve DiAntonio; for cooking dinner and love, Tom Neff; for making life beautiful, Alec and Megan Bartsch.

Contents

The
Color Revolution

When I wrote *Color Me Beautiful* in 1979, I had no idea so many people would buy it. But now, almost 4 million copies later, I know that millions of women needed (as I did) a sensible system for looking great and for pulling together a workable, coordinated, and yes, exciting wardrobe.

It started with a simple idea—that we all have special colors that make us look and feel terrific, colors that are grouped for easy reference into four palettes, based on the seasons of nature. The Winter woman looks great in black and white and bright, primary colors—the sharp contrast of wintertime. Autumn wears the earth tones best; Summer, the soft whites, blues, and blue-greens of a summer day; and Spring, the fresh, new colors of a spring garden.

Less than ten years ago, I was refining the Color Me Beautiful system in my basement, with neighborhood teenagers assembling our color swatches by hand. Today, there are Color Me Beautiful consultants all over the United States and in thirty foreign countries, and the book has been published in seventeen languages. Color Me Beautiful has become a multimillion-dollar company. Why? Because the system works! We've branched out from color and image consultations and now even sell our own cosmetics, fragrances, and clothing.

And it's in large part because of you. *You* carried your color swatches into the stores and insisted on buying *your* colors.

Today, stores, cosmetic companies, and manufacturers are using our seasonal color concept to market their products, which makes shopping easier for all of us. Color Me Beautiful, with your help, created change. We started a color revolution!

Color Me Beautiful has been rewarding for me not only professionally, but also in an even more important way. Thousands of women have written to tell me how finding their colors changed their lives. Some had felt unattractive; some had never had satisfying clothes or a wardrobe that was workable or fun; some had had serious illnesses or accidents and now feel their colors have given them a new lease on life.

It has been thrilling to see the positive impact Color Me Beautiful has had on so many women. And now I've applied the same principles to makeup, to take away the mystery and show you the magic of color so you'll look and feel more beautiful than ever.

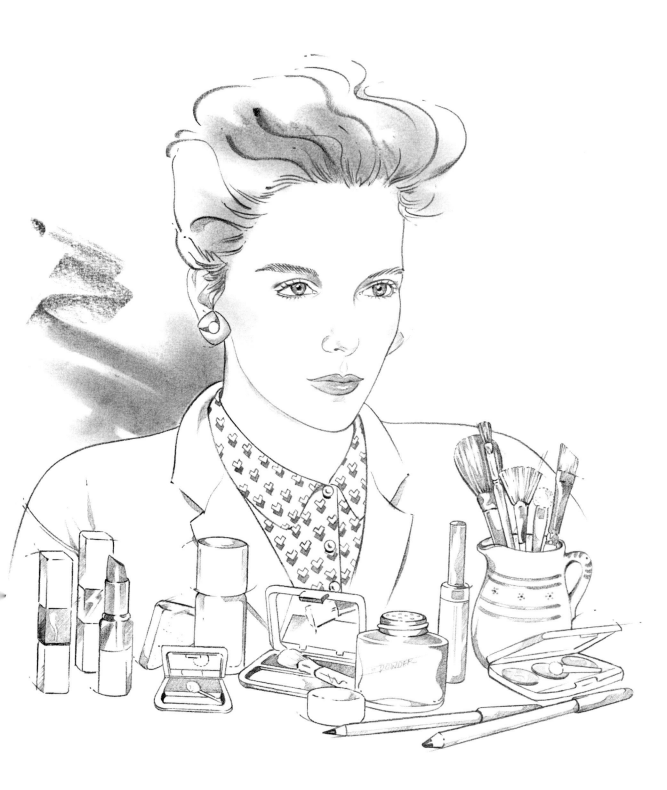

Part I

Color Essentials

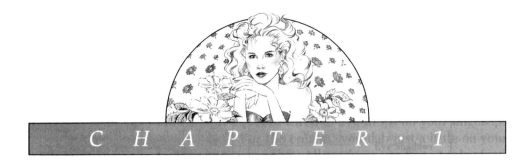

Makeup Magic—

It Works, But How Does It Work for Me?

We all love to see makeovers, don't we? It's intriguing to thumb through a magazine and see a woman with a pale, blotchy face turn into a ravishing beauty on the very same page. And we picture ourselves—in the hands of some fabulous makeup artist—looking gorgeous, too. Or perhaps, just maybe, we could do it ourselves. But how?

As I've traveled the country giving lectures and teaching classes, I've become more convinced than ever that the majority of women are *intimidated* by makeup. These are the comments I frequently hear:

"Where should I put the blush?"
"How much should I put on?"
"What color lipstick should I buy?"
"I don't know how to use a lip pencil."
"My husband thinks makeup looks unnatural."
"How do I put on eye makeup?"
"What color should it be?"

"Won't it make my wrinkles show?"
"Foundation is too thick and gloppy—I don't like the way it feels."
"Powder makes my face look dry and cakey."

I love answering these questions, working with women, and taking the fear out of wearing and applying makeup.

Growing up in Los Angeles, I was surrounded by movie stars and Hollywood's emphasis on beauty. Instruction on applying makeup was available for young girls, and when I was in the ninth grade, my mother took me to a makeup salon to learn how to use cosmetics. The makeup artist showed me how to use a lipstick brush to outline my lips and how to put the lipstick on straight. She also mixed some powder for me. For some reason, perhaps because I was so young, I didn't learn about blush or eye makeup. For several years I wore the lipstick she select- ed for me (peach—a lovely shade for her coloring, but, alas, not for mine), and I would dot lipstick on my cheeks and blend it with my little finger. In college, I finally discovered powdered blush, and somewhere along the line I started using eyeliner and mascara, but I didn't use eye shadow until I was almost thirty.

I shudder to think of the colors I used to wear, but today I am an expert on makeup. I came to my expertise through my years of teaching the principles of Color Me Beautiful, studying with many makeup artists, and experimenting with thousands of women—women with all sizes and shapes of faces and eyes, with young skin and old skin, with complexions and eyes of many different shades.

Most women, I've discovered, have received even less instruction than I did as a young girl. Consequently, many don't wear much makeup, and those who do often apply it incorrectly.

Yet today's women are more up to date than ever. They've read the statistics— women who wear makeup earn 20 percent more than those who don't. And, in spite of what some men say, makeup, naturally applied, attracts them. What men don't like is makeup that shows or looks garish—which often happens when we wear the wrong color.

When we were selecting models for the photographs in *Color Me Beautiful*, dozens of "beautiful" young women appeared with their portfolios. Our young art director was in ecstasy over the gorgeous women we chose. He could hardly wait for the photography shoot so he could gaze at them once more. The morning arrived, and in they came, one after another, each with scraggly straight hair, looking pale and plain with no makeup, wearing jeans and sweatshirts. Robert panicked. "Where are all the pretty ones?" he whispered. "Don't worry. They're here," I replied. Once the makeup artist had worked her magic with the proper colors, her wonderful makeup techniques, and the electric curlers and blow dryer, the beautiful women were indeed there.

We *all* can look beautiful, and no one has to look overly made up to do so. People won't notice your makeup when it is well chosen and properly applied. They will just notice that you are looking better than ever!

When we do a color analysis, my consultant applies the correct makeup colors to her client's face before "draping" her with fabric swatches of the clothing colors that look so beautiful on her. Often, the transformation is dramatic. I have watched the right colors transform women from plain to gorgeous in minutes. The right makeup, applied smoothly and naturally, works magic.

Here are some real-life examples:

Maggie left our class—after looking at herself in the mirror many times—grinning from ear to ear. When she got home, her husband kept mentioning how "happy" and "radiant" she looked that evening. "He never even noticed I had on makeup," she said. "He just said I looked pretty." Maggie's husband liked women to look "natural," so she had never worn makeup before.

Linda's husband had left her. Linda was in her late thirties, one of that generation of women who didn't wear makeup in high school or college because it wasn't in vogue. "Can you believe he left me for an *older* woman?" she said. Linda's morale needed a boost, so we gave her the whole works. She started wearing her colors, got a stylish new haircut, and practiced applying makeup until she got it right. She positively sparkled in her salmon pink blush and lipstick, so perfect for her blond hair and ivory complexion. Linda soon reported that her social life was terrific, and, more importantly, she was excited about her new life.

Oops. Someone goofed. Wendy had already been color analyzed as a Summer when she came to take our makeup class. As she was applying blush and lipstick, it rapidly became apparent that the Summer makeup colors did not look good on her. When she switched to an Autumn shade of lipstick, her face came to life. What a difference! The quickest way to select your season is to try on several shades of lipstick. When the color is *on* your skin, you can immediately see which season's shade is best. Much to Wendy's relief, her Summer wardrobe was not a total loss. Many of the Summer colors she had purchased were similar to Autumn shades—because they were intuitively her favorites. With her new Autumn makeup and a few "right-color" scarves, most of her clothing worked.

The story of Mary is one that touches my heart. Mary had lost her grown daughter in an automobile accident and was still severely depressed after a year. On the advice of her counselor, and in an effort to pull her life together, she came to one of my consultants in the Chicago area. My consultant (bless her) had Mary come into her studio almost every day for three weeks to help her with her makeup. Mary had previously worn only lipstick and blush and had never seen herself looking glamorous before. Gradually, Mary began to think about her own life, and she decided to look for a job that would challenge her. She was hired quickly, and though still grieving, Mary is looking and feeling more beautiful inside and out.

Penny was an extremely attractive woman, already adept at applying makeup. Several weeks after she'd had her colors analyzed and had bought her new makeup, she popped in to see us, looking for all the world like Miss America. "You know, it's just amazing. I remember how I used to feel that my face looked drab, or tired—or something! I'd put on more and more blush, but it just didn't seem to perk me up. Now I realize it was the wrong color. I was wearing tawny peach blush and an earthy brown lipstick, and here I am a Winter, needing pinks and fuchsias. No wonder I felt drab. And think of all the money I wasted!"

Brooke never had a date all through high school. Her mom brought her to one of our color-and-makeup classes, where she learned she was a Summer. Brooke skipped foundation because of her youth, but she loved herself in the soft rose blush and lipstick and the subtle shades of eye shadow she learned to apply. It was inspiring to see how good she felt about herself. She said she had never felt pretty before. Brooke's mom is a friend, so I've kept in touch, and I'm happy to say that Brooke not only has a boyfriend, but also recently won a beauty contest sponsored at her college by a national magazine.

In this book, I will teach you how to choose and apply the perfect makeup for you. In Part I, you'll familiarize yourself with the color essentials. First you'll find your best colors by taking the Color Test. Then I'll show you the full range of makeup colors that complement you. Even if you already know your season, and have enjoyed wearing the right colors before, you may not be fully aware of the variety within your makeup color palette—or how to perfect the harmony of your clothing and makeup combinations. You'll learn to build a "makeup wardrobe," just as you learned to build a clothing wardrobe in *Color Me Beautiful*.

In Part II, you'll get a Color Me Beautiful makeup lesson. I'll lead you step by step through the application of your makeup, just as we do in our Color Me Beautiful makeup classes, from basic skin care to everyday makeup to makeup for special occasions. We'll keep it simple, so that with a little practice you will feel comfortable and satisfied with your makeup. Once you've mastered the techniques, you will be able to apply your basic, everyday, go-to-work look in about six minutes, or spend perhaps ten or fifteen minutes if you want to do something more elaborate for evening.

Finally, in Part III we'll discuss the finishing touches for your Color Me Beautiful look: your hair, your nails, and even your fragrance!

Read the chapters without trying to retain everything. I've summarized all the instructions at the end of the book in a flip chart you can remove. Place it on your vanity or bathroom counter so you can follow the easy instructions page by page. Once you've applied your makeup a number of times, the routine will become second nature—as easy as brushing your teeth.

I hope you will love this book and keep it next to your copy of *Color Me Beautiful*. It's not essential that you read *Color Me Beautiful* before enjoying this book, but if you haven't read it, I suggest you do. It contains a thorough explanation of the color system and how to determine your personal colors, as well as valuable information on your wardrobe, style, figure, and hair. The principles of the Color Me Beautiful system are timeless, so nothing you learn from either book will go out of style. You can always adapt a fashion trend to your best look. So enjoy yourself, and have fun looking more beautiful than ever.

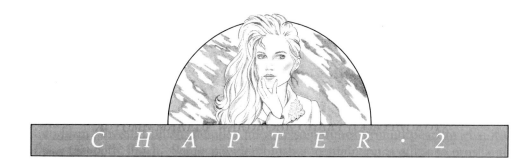

Color Me Beautiful: The Palettes

The first step in using makeup to your greatest advantage is finding the right colors! The wrong color on your face can look worse than no makeup at all—and the most expert application in the world cannot compensate for an unflattering color.

Color Me Beautiful uses the names of the seasons of nature as a way of describing your coloring and the colors that most flatter you. You are called a Winter, Summer, Autumn, or Spring, depending on the color of your skin, hair, and eyes. Each season's palette contains its own special array of colors, and *your* coloring is in harmony with *one* of them. Both your makeup and your clothing colors derive from your season's palette.

We all have genetically inherited coloring: skin tone, eye color, hair color. Looking around any room full of people you can see the varieties of skin tones. It is impossible for the same shades of makeup to look terrific on all these skin tones. That's why a hot, fashion color can't look good on everyone. We need colors that complement, rather than clash with, our skin.

Winter women look their most beautiful in makeup of sparkling pinks and reds, with cool eye shadows in charcoal, blues, and purples. Their wardrobe colors are the jewel tones and the dramatic black and white of wintertime. Summers are flattered by makeup in soft, gentle pinks, mauves, and watermelons, with eye shadows in hazy grape, aqua, and azure—shades of summer. The Summer woman's wardrobe contains cool, soft colors ranging from pastel pinks and blues to deep, dusty shades of plum, fuchsia, and spruce.

Autumns radiate in the rich, warm tones of fall. In makeup or wardrobe, their elegance shines in shades of coppery reds, tawny peach, and earthy shades of green, brown, and teal. The Spring woman comes to life in the clear, warm colors of springtime. Her lips delight in coral pinks, peaches, and luscious poppy reds, while her eyes are flattered by soft golden browns, greens, and aquas. Spring's wardrobe contains the colors of a vibrant spring bouquet—yellow, pink, periwinkle blue, coral, and fresh greens.

To determine your best colors, you need to analyze your coloring—your skin, hair, and eyes. If you have already read *Color Me Beautiful* or have had your colors analyzed by a professional color consultant, then you're familiar with your season's palette. If you don't know your season, you'll have a chance to take the Color Test in Chapter 3. For now, just look at the color palettes to familiarize yourself with them. In this chapter, I'll describe the makeup color palette appropriate for each season and will review the palettes for wardrobe colors.

THE SEASONAL PALETTES: MAKEUP

Makeup colors come in both *cool* and *warm* shades. Cool shades are ones that have a blue or gray undertone; warm shades have a yellow or golden undertone.

Winter and Summer are the cool seasons. Look at their makeup palettes on pages 21 and 23. Notice that the lipstick and blush colors are in tones of rose, blue-pink, fuchsia, plum, and burgundy. The red lipsticks are bluish, rather than orangish.

The eye shadows, too, include cool colors: gray-blues and navies, grape and purple, gray, pink, lavender, mint and spruce green, as well as soft white, grayish browns, and silver. There are no oranges, peaches, or golden colors in the cool makeup palettes. Warm colors will not be flattering on the Winter or Summer woman!

Now study the warm Autumn and Spring palettes on pages 25 and 27. See how these palettes contain warm lipstick and blush shades of peach, coral, and orange. Here the reds have an orange tone. Even the pinks in the Spring palette are warm pinks—containing yellow. Compare them to the blue-pinks on the Winter and Summer pages. Notice, too, that the eye shadows consist of tones of peach, gold, golden greens, honey, and coppery browns, as well as copper, bronze, and gold. There are no blue-based colors on the Autumn and Spring charts, for they will be harsh and aging on a warm skin tone. They will actually clash with your coloring and look unharmonious and unattractive.

In general, when selecting makeup colors your first concern is whether you are warm or cool. Summers and Winters can share some of the same makeup shades, as can Autumns and Springs. Spruce green and cocoa eye shadow, for example, flatter both Winters and Summers, even though the Winter woman wears a brighter pine green or a deep black/brown in clothing. Sage green eye shadow complements both Autumn and Spring eyes, although only Autumn wears it in clothing.

You will undoubtedly notice that a few eye shadow colors show up on all four charts: champagne, aqua, teal blue, teal green, and periwinkle blue. These shades are on the borderline of warm and cool, and will complement both types of skin tone. In addition, you will notice that your makeup choices include color names that are not on the wardrobe charts. Cosmetic colors blend into your skin and allow you more options.

Next, look at the charts for what I call *value*—how light or dark the colors are. Note that the Winter and Autumn charts contain deeper and brighter colors.

Winter and Autumn women, in general, have darker hair and eyes, and need richer colors to offset their coloring. Spring and Summer women often have lighter hair and fairer complexions than their Winter and Autumn counterparts. Their makeup colors will always be lighter, ranging from very soft to medium bright.

Last, note the *clarity* of the colors—whether they are muted down or clear. Both Winter and Spring women look best in makeup colors that are fairly clear and vibrant, even though Winter's are darker than Spring's. See how the lipstick and blush colors are perky and lively. Spring has many soft shades, but they are clear, not dusty. Autumn and Summer women can wear both clear and muted colors, but are often best in the dusty ones. See how Autumn's red is a brick shade—a muted red. Summer's pink is a dusty rose. Even though all eye shadows have to be somewhat toned down to look natural, you will still find that Summer is best in a grayish grape while Winter chooses a clearer purple. Autumn can wear a smoky turquoise, but Spring needs a clearer aqua.

Your makeup palette contains all the colors you will need to complement the entire spectrum of your season's wardrobe. In addition, the colors in your makeup palette automatically blend beautifully with each other—because they derive from the same cool or warm base. You will delight in the variety of colors and creative combinations in your palette, and in the confidence of knowing that the colors all harmonize with *you*!

THE SEASONAL PALETTES: WARDROBE REVIEW

Like your makeup, your wardrobe palettes also exhibit three distinct qualities: color (warm or cool), value (light or dark), and clarity (clear or muted).

Look at the color bars on pages 28, 29, 30, and 31, which depict the wardrobe colors for each season. The Winter and Summer palettes are cool, while Autumn's and Spring's are warm. Note that Winter and Summer both have blue-reds, blue-greens, and blue-based pinks such as fuchsia, magenta, and rose. The

Autumn and Spring palettes contain yellow-greens, orange-reds, and golden browns and yellows—all warm colors.

Autumn and Winter colors are again the deepest and most full-bodied, while Summer and Spring have many pastels and light to medium shades. Notice that Winter and Autumn have colors such as black, dark brown, burgundy, mahogany, pine green, forest green, and purple, compared to the powder pink, peach, lavender, sky blue, soft fuchsia, and light orange found in the Summer or Spring palettes.

Last, examine the clarity of the wardrobe colors. The Winter and Spring palettes contain only clear colors; Autumn and Summer colors are more muted.

The following charts list by name the wardrobe colors for each season, in the same order as they appear on the color bars. You'll find a few new colors, ones that were not included in the original *Color Me Beautiful* book. Because the color bars on pages 28, 29, 30, and 31 are small, and because printed color is not as true as colored fabric, you may want to acquire a set of fabric swatches in your season's wardrobe colors to use as a shopping guide. The same colors can be used to help select makeup shades. At the back of the book I've included information on how to obtain fabric swatches.

WINTER WARDROBE COLORS

The Winter woman is best in clear colors and sharp contrast. She wears black and white well and looks great in true, primary colors, royal shades, and ice colors. She avoids golden browns, orange, gold, and dusty pastels.

Neutrals: for coats, suits, jackets, pants, basic dresses

Navy	Light True Gray
Black	Black-Brown
Charcoal Gray	Taupe (Gray Beige)
Medium True Gray	

Lights: for blouses, lingerie, evening wear, warm-weather attire

Pure White	Icy Pink
Icy Gray	Icy Green
Icy Blue	Icy Violet
Icy Yellow	Icy Aqua

Basic and Bright/Accent Colors: for blouses, sweaters, sportswear, dresses (can also be worn in pants, jackets, and skirts)

Royal Blue	Royal Purple
True Blue	Fuchsia
Bright Periwinkle Blue	Magenta
Pine Green	Deep Hot Pink
Emerald Green	Shocking Pink
True Green	Clear Teal
Light True Green	Chinese Blue
Vivid Cranberry	Hot Turquoise
Bright Burgundy	Bright Emerald Turquoise
Blue-Red	Lemon Yellow
True Red	

Black-brown, dark periwinkle blue, vivid cranberry, clear teal, and bright emerald turquoise are new additions to the Winter palette.

SUMMER WARDROBE COLORS

The Summer woman thrives on gentle, cool colors, slightly muted, from pastel to deep. She dresses with soft contrast, never sharp or harsh. Summer avoids golden tones, orange, black, stark white, and extremely bright, clear colors.

Neutrals: for coats, suits, jackets, pants, basic dresses

Grayed Navy	Light Blue Gray
Grayed Blue	Rose Brown
Charcoal Blue Gray	Cocoa

Lights: for blouses, lingerie, evening wear, warm-weather attire

Soft White	Powder Pink
Rose Beige	Light Mauve
Powder Blue	Lavender
Light Lemon Yellow	

Basic and Bright/Accent Colors: for blouses, sweaters, sportswear, dresses (can also be worn in pants, jackets, and skirts)

Periwinkle Blue	Rose Pink
Sky Blue	Deep Rose
Medium Blue	Blue-Red
Cadet Blue	Watermelon Red
Pastel Aqua	Burgundy/Maroon
Medium Aqua	Mauve
Soft Teal	Raspberry
Pastel Blue-Green	Orchid
Medium Blue-Green	Soft Fuchsia
Deep Blue-Green	Medium Violet
Spruce Green	Plum
Pastel Pink	

Cadet blue, medium aqua, soft teal, spruce green, and medium violet are new additions to the Summer palette.

AUTUMN WARDROBE COLORS

The Autumn woman looks best in warm, earthy colors, ranging from medium to dark. Her colors must always have a rich quality, even in the lighter shades. She avoids all blue-based colors, fuchsias, blue-pinks, and silvery grays, as well as black and pure white.

Neutrals: for coats, suits, jackets, pants, basic dresses

Dark Brown/Charcoal	Olive Green
Coffee Brown	Grayed Green
Khaki/Tan	Marine Navy
Camel	Warm Gray/Pewter

Lights: for blouses, lingerie, evening wear, warm-weather attire

Oyster White	Light Peach/Apricot
Warm Beige	Light Periwinkle Blue
Light Gold/Buff	

Basic and Bright/Accent Colors: for blouses, sweaters, sportswear, dresses (can also be worn in pants, jackets, and skirts)

Deep Periwinkle Blue	Mustard
Purple	Terra Cotta
Aubergine/Eggplant	Orange/Pumpkin
Medium Warm Bronze	Orange-Red/Bittersweet
Forest Green	Dark Tomato Red
Bright Yellow-Green	Brown Burgundy
Jade Green	Rust
Turquoise	Mahogany
Teal Blue	Deep Peach/Apricot
Golden Yellow	Salmon
Gold	Salmon Pink

Khaki/tan, marine navy, warm gray/pewter, light gold/buff, light peach/apricot, light periwinkle blue, purple, aubergine/eggplant, and salmon pink are new additions to the Autumn palette.

SPRING WARDROBE COLORS

Spring women look best in warm, clear colors, ranging from pastel to medium bright. They wear crisp contrast well. Springs avoid dark, harsh colors, as well as blue-based pinks, reds, and grays.

Neutrals: for coats, suits, jackets, pants, basic dresses

Clear Bright Navy
Medium Warm Gray
Light Warm Gray
Chocolate Brown

Medium Golden Brown
Camel/Golden Tan
Light Warm Beige

Lights: for blouses, lingerie, evening wear, warm-weather attire

Ivory
Buff
Light Peach/Apricot

Warm Pastel Pink
Light Blue/Periwinkle

Basic and Bright/Accent Colors: for blouses, sweaters, sportswear, dresses (can also be worn in pants, jackets, and skirts)

Light Clear Navy
Light True Blue
Medium Blue
Periwinkle Blue
Dark Periwinkle Blue
Medium Violet
Pastel Yellow-Green
Bright Yellow-Green
Light True Green
Kelly Green
Coral Pink
Clear Bright Warm Pink

Peach/Apricot
Clear Salmon
Bright Coral
Light Orange
Orange-Red
Clear Bright Red
Light Warm Aqua
Clear Bright Aqua
Light Teal Blue
Emerald Turquoise
Light Clear Gold
Bright Golden Yellow

Clear bright navy, medium warm gray, chocolate brown, buff, light blue/periwinkle, and light teal blue are new additions to the Spring palette.

The following pictures show you women of each seasonal type, in right and wrong makeup colors, along with the appropriate makeup palette. You can see how well the correct colors complement the coloring of the models. Once you have determined your colors, you can use your season's makeup chart as a shopping guide. Since cosmetic manufacturers can call a color anything they want, your color chart will help you get started. I've given the colors descriptive names to further assist you, as it is difficult to print makeup colors accurately on paper. Don't feel you need to own *all* these colors. Rather, the chart represents your *range* of choices. If you are fair, you'll choose the lighter shades; if your coloring is vivid, you'll wear brighter shades.

The pictures also show you some of the common mistakes women make in applying their makeup so you can see what a difference it makes to place the colors correctly. The last pages feature eye makeup on several different eye shapes and colors, to help you understand how to make up your own eyes.

The first model is shown three ways: with no makeup, with minimal makeup, and with complete makeup, adding foundation, powder, and eye makeup. I urge *you* to go for the complete, finished look. A dash of hurriedly applied blush and lipstick is OK for the tennis court, but for the rest of life, it's not enough. Whether at the office, a party, or among friends and family, you're cheating yourself from looking your beautiful best if you don't take the few minutes it requires each morning to achieve a natural but "complete" look. You'll look more polished, more elegant, more professional, and you'll feel better about yourself, too. You deserve all the compliments that will come your way!

THE COMPLETE LOOK

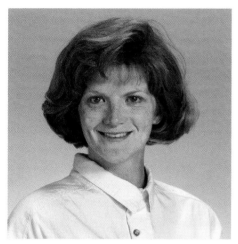

*L*ook at the difference in Autumn Jennifer with and without makeup! Imagine Jennifer applying for an important job with no makeup on. But note, too, the difference when Jennifer applies only lipstick, blush and mascara, in the minimal picture. Even though her hair is done and she's donned her earrings, her look doesn't compare to the polished image she creates by adding foundation, powder, eye shadow, liner, and brow definer. Add a scarf and necklace, too, and Jennifer has really completed her look.

NO MAKEUP

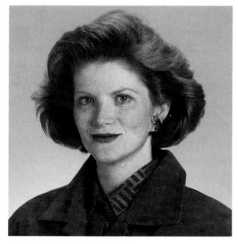

MINIMAL MAKEUP

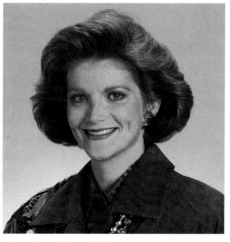

COMPLETE LOOK

WINTER

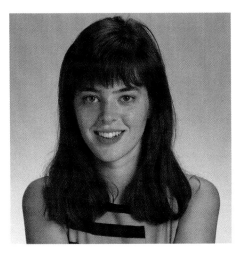

NO MAKEUP

*D*iane is a Winter, with light, neutral beige skin, gray-green eyes, and dark ash brown hair. Even though she is a beautiful girl, Diane's skin looks dull in the pumpkin-colored blouse and orange makeup tones. In addition, Diane has applied her blush too low, too far forward, and too heavily— a common makeup mistake. See how Diane radiates in her cool-tone royal blue blouse, hot pink lipstick, pink blush, and silver, lavender, and purple eye shadows. Her blush lightly dusts the apple of her cheek, blending towards the upper half of her ear.

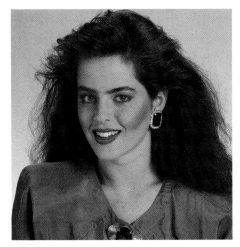

WRONG

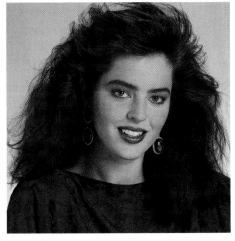

RIGHT

WINTER MAKEUP PALETTE

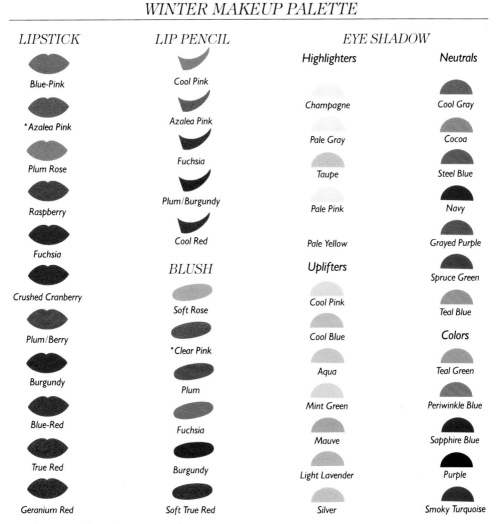

LIPSTICK

Blue-Pink

*Azalea Pink

Plum Rose

Raspberry

Fuchsia

Crushed Cranberry

Plum/Berry

Burgundy

Blue-Red

True Red

Geranium Red

LIP PENCIL

Cool Pink

Azalea Pink

Fuchsia

Plum/Burgundy

Cool Red

BLUSH

Soft Rose

*Clear Pink

Plum

Fuchsia

Burgundy

Soft True Red

EYE SHADOW

Highlighters

Champagne

Pale Gray

Taupe

Pale Pink

Pale Yellow

Uplifters

Cool Pink

Cool Blue

Aqua

Mint Green

Mauve

Light Lavender

Silver

Neutrals

Cool Gray

Cocoa

Steel Blue

Navy

Grayed Purple

Spruce Green

Teal Blue

Colors

Teal Green

Periwinkle Blue

Sapphire Blue

Purple

Smoky Turquoise

Foundations: Sand, Cool Beige, Neutral Beige, Rose Beige, Deep Rose Beige, Rose Brown
Basic Mascara: Black, Black-Brown, Navy, Spruce Green
Eyeliner: Black, Charcoal Gray, Navy, Spruce Green, Teal Blue, Steel Blue, Deep Purple, Periwinkle Blue
*Best test colors.

SUMMER

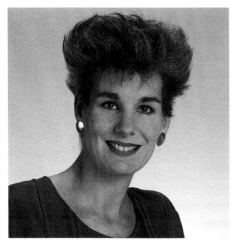

NO MAKEUP

*S*ummer Nancy has pink-beige skin, gray-blue eyes, and soft salt-and-peppery hair. See how she glows in her correct colors and makeup. Her pink blouse enhances her beauty, as does her lightly frosted rose lipstick, rose blush, and pink, gray, and steel blue eyeshadows. In the apricot blouse and makeup, Nancy looks sallow. Note especially the difference in eye makeup. In the "wrong" picture, Nancy has applied dark teal eyeshadow to her lids and yellow highlighter on her brow area—exactly the wrong application technique for her eyes. Because Nancy's lids don't show and she has a large brow area, her eyes are more complemented by applying a light shade to the lid, and a medium shade to her orbital bone, as in the "right" picture.

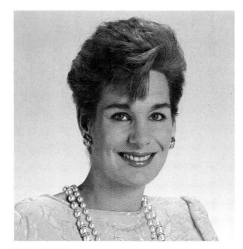

WRONG

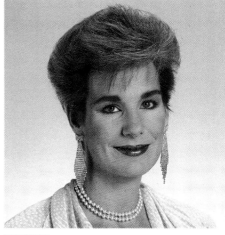

RIGHT

SUMMER MAKEUP PALETTE

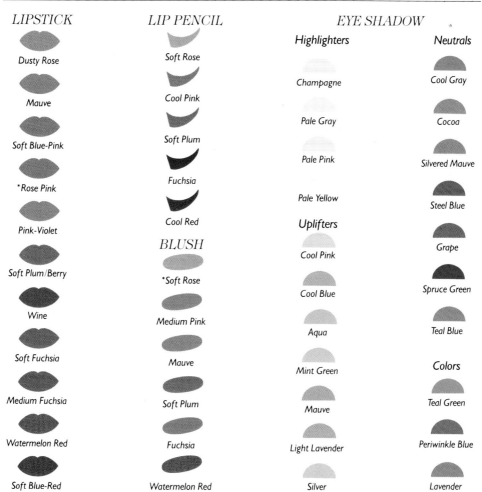

LIPSTICK

Dusty Rose

Mauve

Soft Blue-Pink

*Rose Pink

Pink-Violet

Soft Plum/Berry

Wine

Soft Fuchsia

Medium Fuchsia

Watermelon Red

Soft Blue-Red

LIP PENCIL

Soft Rose

Cool Pink

Soft Plum

Fuchsia

Cool Red

BLUSH

*Soft Rose

Medium Pink

Mauve

Soft Plum

Fuchsia

Watermelon Red

EYE SHADOW

Highlighters

Champagne

Pale Gray

Pale Pink

Pale Yellow

Uplifters

Cool Pink

Cool Blue

Aqua

Mint Green

Mauve

Light Lavender

Silver

Neutrals

Cool Gray

Cocoa

Silvered Mauve

Steel Blue

Grape

Spruce Green

Teal Blue

Colors

Teal Green

Periwinkle Blue

Lavender

Foundations: Pale Pink Beige, Cool Beige, Pink Beige, Neutral Beige, Deep Rose Beige, Rose Brown
Basic Mascara: Brown-Black, Brown, Navy, Spruce Green
Eyeliner: Charcoal, Medium Gray, Taupe Brown, Spruce Green, Teal Blue, Navy, Slate Blue, Amethyst,
        Periwinkle Blue

*Best test colors.

AUTUMN

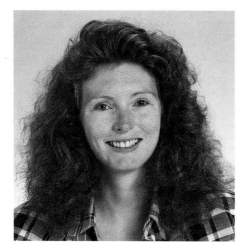

NO MAKEUP

Sharon has typical Autumn coloring: ivory skin, red hair and yellow-green eyes. Doesn't she look gorgeous in her forest green and orange-red clothing combination, with orange lipstick, peach blush, and gold, peach, and brown tones on her eyes. See how her eyes sparkle. Even though fashionably dressed in black and burgundy, Sharon looks harsh when she wears these cool colors and burgundy makeup tones. Further, Sharon has made the mistake of lining her lips with a burgundy lip pencil that shows, making her lips look unnatural and severe. See how much softer she looks in her correct colors and more natural application of makeup.

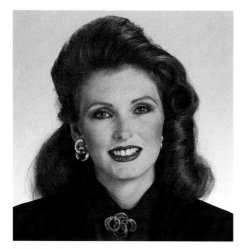

WRONG

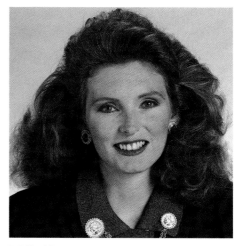

RIGHT

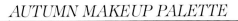

AUTUMN MAKEUP PALETTE

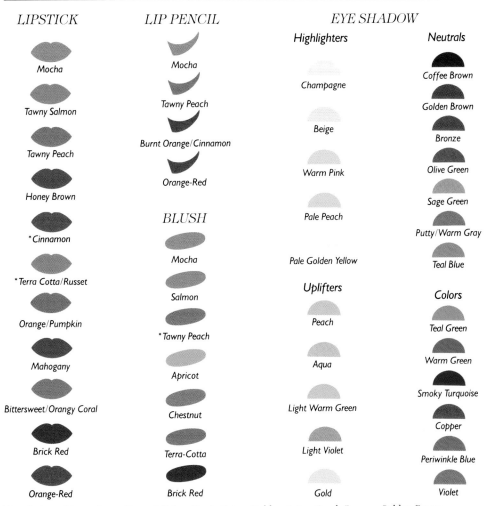

LIPSTICK

Mocha

Tawny Salmon

Tawny Peach

Honey Brown

*Cinnamon

*Terra Cotta/Russet

Orange/Pumpkin

Mahogany

Bittersweet/Orangy Coral

Brick Red

Orange-Red

LIP PENCIL

Mocha

Tawny Peach

Burnt Orange/Cinnamon

Orange-Red

BLUSH

Mocha

Salmon

*Tawny Peach

Apricot

Chestnut

Terra-Cotta

Brick Red

EYE SHADOW

Highlighters

Champagne

Beige

Warm Pink

Pale Peach

Pale Golden Yellow

Uplifters

Peach

Aqua

Light Warm Green

Light Violet

Gold

Neutrals

Coffee Brown

Golden Brown

Bronze

Olive Green

Sage Green

Putty/Warm Gray

Teal Blue

Colors

Teal Green

Warm Green

Smoky Turquoise

Copper

Periwinkle Blue

Violet

Foundations: Bisque, Ivory, Natural Beige, Peach Beige, Golden Beige, Peach Bronze, Golden Brown
Basic Mascara: Black, Black-Brown, Navy, Olive Green
Eyeliner: Brown, Olive Green, Forest Green, Teal Blue, Marine Navy, Teal Green, Violet, Turquoise
*Best test colors.

25

SPRING

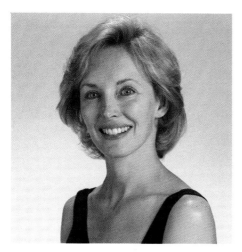

NO MAKEUP

*J*ill is a Spring with a delicate ivory skin tone, teal blue eyes and flaxen blonde hair. Her fair coloring is overpowered by the cool, dark red in her dress and lipstick, and the heavy, solid line of black eyeliner. In her orange-red suit, with soft poppy red lipstick and blush, a subtle, smudgy eyeliner of medium brown, and pale eye shadow shades of champagne, peach, and brown, Jill looks young, fresh, and beautiful.

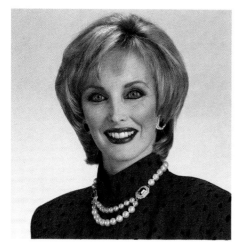

WRONG

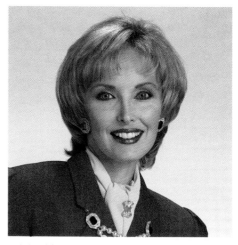

RIGHT

SPRING MAKEUP PALETTE

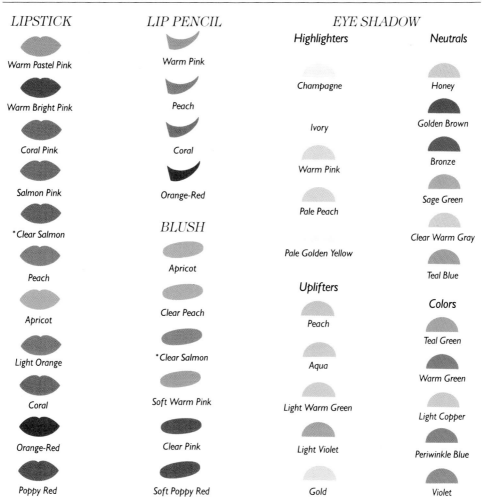

LIPSTICK

Warm Pastel Pink

Warm Bright Pink

Coral Pink

Salmon Pink

*Clear Salmon

Peach

Apricot

Light Orange

Coral

Orange-Red

Poppy Red

LIP PENCIL

Warm Pink

Peach

Coral

Orange-Red

BLUSH

Apricot

Clear Peach

*Clear Salmon

Soft Warm Pink

Clear Pink

Soft Poppy Red

EYE SHADOW

Highlighters

Champagne

Ivory

Warm Pink

Pale Peach

Pale Golden Yellow

Uplifters

Peach

Aqua

Light Warm Green

Light Violet

Gold

Neutrals

Honey

Golden Brown

Bronze

Sage Green

Clear Warm Gray

Teal Blue

Colors

Teal Green

Warm Green

Light Copper

Periwinkle Blue

Violet

Foundations: Porcelain, Ivory, Peach, Peach Beige, Golden Beige, Golden Bronze
Basic Mascara: Brown-Black, Brown, Navy, Olive Green
Eyeliner: Brown, Olive Green, Sage Green, Teal Blue, Teal Green, Turquoise, Violet, Slate Blue, Periwinkle Blue
*Best test colors.

WINTER MAKEUP WARDROBE

PINK

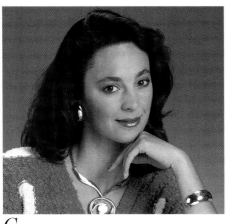

*C*asual: pink lips and cheeks; eyeliner, gray; eye shadows, champagne, pink, teal.

FUCHSIA

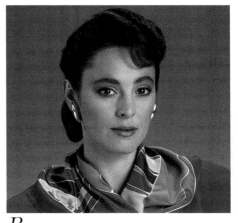

*B*usiness: fuchsia lips and cheeks; eyeliner, forest green and charcoal gray; eye shadows, pink, purple, and spruce green.

TRUE RED

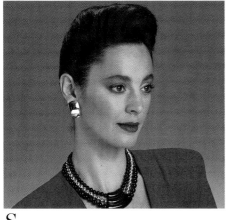

*S*ophisticated: true red lips and soft red cheeks; charcoal gray eyeliner; silver and gray eye shadows.

BURGUNDY

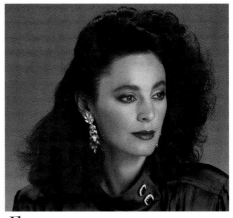

*E*vening. burgundy lips and cheeks; smudged black eyeliner; silver, gray, and sapphire blue eye shadows.

*D*oreen has typical Winter coloring: light olive skin, dark brown eyes, and black-brown hair. She looks wonderful in all the cool, vivid colors of the Winter palette.

SUMMER MAKEUP WARDROBE

WATERMELON RED

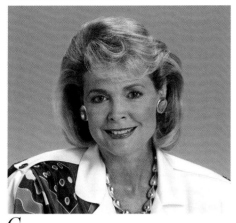

*C*asual: watermelon red lips and cheeks; slate blue eyeliner; champagne and cool blue eye shadows.

SOFT FUCHSIA

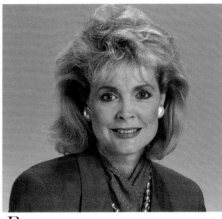

*B*usiness: Soft fuchsia lips and cheeks; taupe brown eyeliner; mauve, cocoa, and grape eye shadows.

BLUE-PINK

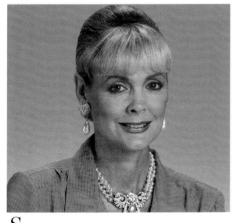

*S*ophisticated: blue-pink lips and rose pink blush; charcoal eyeliner; pink, cool gray, and teal green eye shadows.

DUSTY ROSE

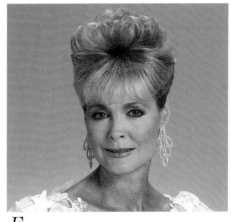

*E*vening: dusty rose lips and rose pink blush; charcoal eyeliner; pink, silver, and lavender eye shadows.

*S*ummer Barbara has rosy beige skin, ash blonde hair and cool blue eyes. Barbara's soft coloring is enhanced by the pinks, blues, and blue-greens of her Summer palette.

29

AUTUMN MAKEUP WARDROBE

ORANGE-RED

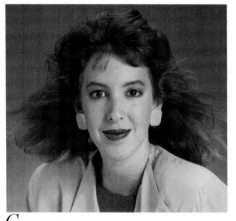

*C*asual: orange-red lips and terra-cotta cheeks; brown eyeliner; golden yellow and brown eye shadows.

HONEY BROWN

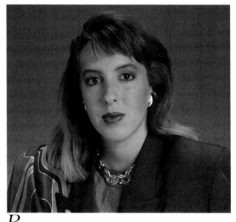

*B*usiness: honey brown lips; chestnut cheeks; brown eyeliner; champagne, bronze, and a hint of teal blue eye shadows.

BRICK RED

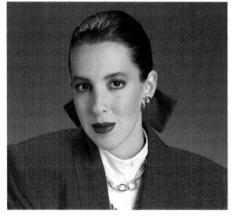

*S*ophisticated: brick red lips and cheeks; brown eyeliner; beige, putty, and coffee brown eye shadows.

CINNAMON

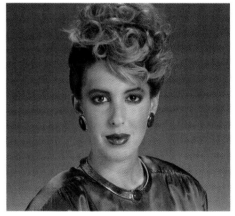

*E*vening: cinnamon lips and apricot cheeks; brown eyeliner and brown kohl pencil lining inner rim of lower lid; peach, gold, and copper eye shadows.

*M*egan's golden coloring is typical of Autumn. Her peach skin tone, dark golden brown eyes and honey hair are complemented by the rich, warm tones of Autumn's palette.

SPRING MAKEUP WARDROBE

CLEAR SALMON

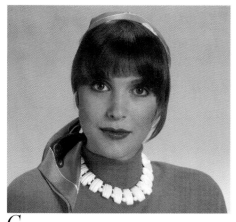

*C*asual: clear salmon lips and cheeks; soft brown eyeliner; brown and peach eye shadows.

ORANGE-RED

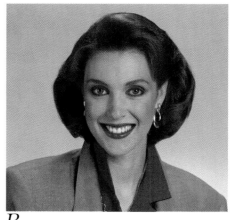

*B*usiness: orange-red lips; poppy red cheeks; ivory, golden brown, and teal eye shadows.

WARM BRIGHT PINK

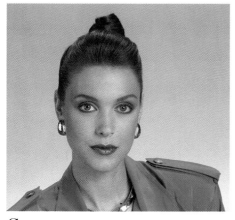

*S*ophisticated: warm pink lips and cheeks; brown and teal blue eyeliners; warm pink, honey, and teal blue eye shadows.

PEACH

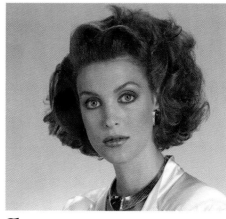

*E*vening: peach lips and cheeks; brown eyeliner; ivory, light violet, and bronze eye shadows.

*R*ebecca's creamy peach skin tone, blue eyes, and golden brown hair are true Spring qualities. Rebecca radiates in her Spring palette of warm, clear colors.

EYE SHAPES

PROPORTIONED LID AND BROW

Example: Spring blue eye

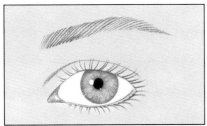

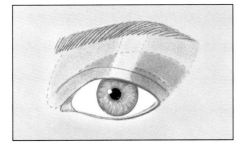

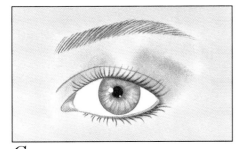

Cover the entire area with highlighter. Then, apply a contour shade to the orbital bone, a deeper shade to the outer corner of the lid, a pale shade to the inner lid, and for evening, a vertical stripe of uplifter above the iris.

LARGE LID; SMALL BROW

Example: Autumn green eye

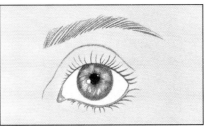

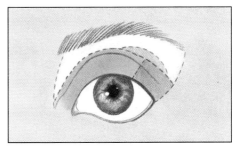

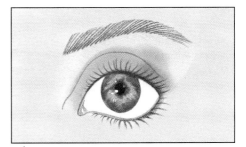

Apply a medium neutral shade to the entire lid, and accentuate the corner of the lid with a deeper shade. Apply a highlighter to the brow area; then, sweep the deeper shade from the outer corner up onto the orbital bone. Finally, apply an uplifter to the crest of the orbital bone.

EYE SHAPES

SMALL LID; LARGE BROW

Example: Summer blue eye

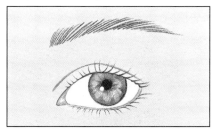

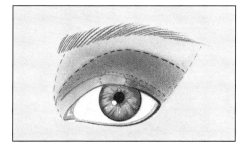

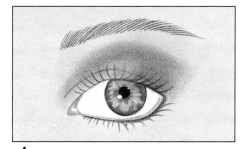

SMALL LID; SMALL BROW

Example: Winter brown eye

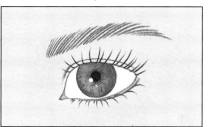

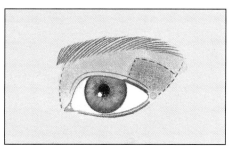

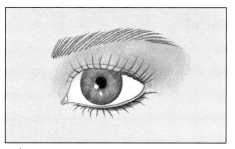

*A*pply highlighter to the entire area and then a darker shade on the orbital bone, bringing it high in the center. Accentuate the outer corner of the eye with a deep shadow, and bring out the lid with a touch of pale color above the iris.

*A*pply a pale color from lashes to brow. Contour the corner with a deeper shade on the outer third of the lid, swept slightly up toward the outer half of the eyebrow. Do not contour the orbital bone.

CHOOSING EYE SHADOW COLORS

RIGHT   WRONG

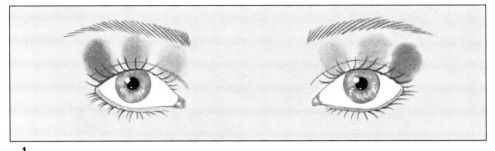

A cool blue eye is enhanced by a similar shade of blue eye shadow but clashes with teal blue shadow, even though the highlighter is correct (as in all the examples).

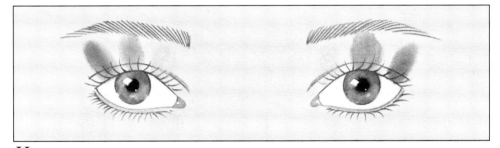

*Y*ellow-green eyes stand out with champagne highlighter and warm, yellow-green eye shadows but recede and look clownish with blue-green eye shadow.

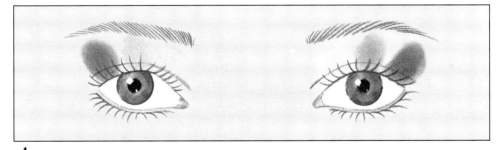

A golden brown eye looks best with golden brown and beige shadows but clashes with rose-brown eye shadow.

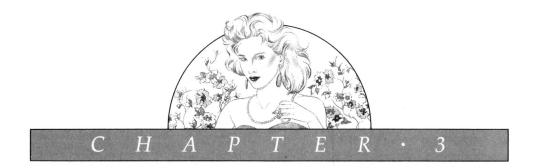

The
Color Test

Determining your colors is easiest with cosmetics! Trying on blush and lipstick colors will quickly show you whether you are a Winter, Summer, Autumn, or Spring.

I've divided the Color Test into two steps. In Step 1, you'll read the descriptions of each seasonal type and select the one or two that best describe you. In Step 2, you'll try on specific makeup colors and compare them. For this you'll need to go to a department store or a drugstore that carries cosmetics tester units so you can have access to many colors.

STEP 1: SELECTING THE DESCRIPTION THAT FITS YOU

As you read these descriptions, recall in your mind several outfits—past or present—that you felt terrific wearing. Did they bring you compliments? Now select the season that best describes you.

WINTER

Clothing: The Winter woman looks best in clear, pure cool colors, ranging from bright to dark pinks, blues, greens, purples, blue-reds, and true reds—the jewel tones. She wears dark, blue-based colors such as navy blue well, and she sparkles in black and white. A Winter doesn't look wonderful in earth tones or any muted colors. She needs brightness and clarity. Even her light colors must be clear and icy, almost like wearing white. She does not enjoy wearing pastels because they don't "do anything" for her. The Winter woman loves to wear red.

Makeup: Winter's best face colors are pink or burgundy blushes and medium to bright pink or fuchsia lipstick as well as true red or burgundy shades. Because she looks best in clear colors she often prefers a slightly frosted lip color. The Winter woman will look drab in brown, rust, or cinnamon lipsticks, and orange or peach shades will make her look sallow (yellow). If she wears a lipstick that is too pale she will look washed out. She needs color!

Coloring: Winter usually has intense coloring: medium to dark hair and deep eye color. Only rarely—very rarely—is she a natural blonde as an adult. Her skin is either very white, dark (black, brown, light brown), olive, gray beige, or neutral beige. A few Winters have rosy cheeks, but most have no visible pink in their skin tone.

The most common Winter types have the following hair, eye color, and skin tone combinations.

Pick out the combination that best describes you, starting with your hair color.

HAIR	EYES	SKIN
Black Dark brown Light blond (rare)	Blue with white flecks	White Rose beige
Black Medium to dark brown	Dark brown	Olive Neutral beige Brown Black
Brown	Hazel (brown/green)	Olive Neutral beige
Brown	Green with white flecks	Neutral beige Gray beige
Salt and pepper Silver gray Pure white	Any of the above	Any of the above

Winter Women: Elizabeth Taylor, Jackie Onassis, Linda Carter, Gloria Vanderbilt, Jaclyn Smith, Linda Ronstadt.

SUMMER

Clothing: The Summer woman has softer coloring than Winter—lighter hair and eye color—and therefore wears less intense colors. She is flattered by pastel to medium-bright blues, pinks, soft fuchsias, blue-greens, lavenders, mauves, and aquas as well as shades of watermelon and blue-reds—all *cool* colors. She wears muted colors such as powder blue or cadet blue well. Any dark color must be grayed down or softened a bit. She is overwhelmed by extremely bright, clear colors. Like Winter, she avoids warm, golden colors, as these will make her face look tired or drawn.

Makeup: Summer's best blush is soft rose or plum, and she glows in lipstick shades of rose pink, light to medium pink or fuchsia, and soft berry colors. Red lipstick is too bright for Summer unless it is a soft watermelon shade. Any orange or peach shades of lipstick or blush will look "brassy," and rust, cinnamon, or brownish shades will look dull.

Coloring: The Summer is often blond as a child, but as she matures her hair darkens to a "dirty" blond or an ashen brunette. A few Summers remain platinum blond. Although never a redhead, some brunette Summers will have purplish red highlights in their hair. Summer's eyes are most often a cool blue or a gray blue, while a few Summers have green eyes, often mixed with brown. A brown-eyed Summer is a rarity indeed, except on a black or Asian woman. (Brown-eyed blondes are usually Autumns.) Summer women often have pinkish skin or a little pinkness in their cheeks. Some, however, have pale beige, very light olive, or translucent "white" skin. Black Summers have light skin (but not golden), and Asian Summers have pale gray beige skin.

The most common combinations of hair, eye color, and skin tone for summer women are:

HAIR	EYES	SKIN
Light to medium brown	Blue with white flecks Hazel (blue/brown) Hazel (green/brown)	White with pale pink cheeks Pinky beige Beige with pink cheeks
Dark blond (ash) Platinum blond	Blue Gray-blue Green with white flecks	Light olive Neutral beige Pinky beige
Dark brown	Blue with white flecks	Pale with pink cheeks Slightly ruddy
Soft salt and pepper Pearl gray Pearl white	Any of the above	Any of the above
Black Charcoal brown	Brown	Light black Light beige (Asian)

Summer Women: Grace Kelly, Farrah Fawcett, Linda Evans, Candace Bergen, Bo Derek.

AUTUMN

Clothing: The Autumn woman loves to wear rich, *warm* colors such as teal blue, bittersweet red, forest green, jade, deep salmon and peach, and coffee brown as well as earthy, muted tones of olive, rust, gold, terra cotta, mustard, and khaki. She looks great in monochromatic outfits of beige and oyster or beige and brown, with lots of gold, brass, or copper jewelry to add warmth and richness. She usually wears muted colors better than clear colors. Even her bright colors are more flattering if they are slightly toned down. Autumns come in two varieties: light-haired ones who tend to prefer soft, earthy, neutral colors, and dark-eyed, dark-haired brunettes, and red heads who love their red, forest, and brighter colors. All Autumns avoid fuchsia, blue-reds, gray, and most pinks because they clash with their golden coloring. Most pale colors, especially blues and pinks, make them look washed out. Autumn women need rich colors!

Makeup: The Autumn woman looks terrific in all the cinnamon, peach, russet, and terra cotta shades of blush and lipstick. Lighter Autumns love mocha and tawny peach lipsticks, while darker Autumns look better in more intense shades of terra cotta or brick red. A pink or fuchsia lipstick will look harsh, even garish, on an Autumn's face.

Coloring: The Autumn woman has hair with red or gold highlights. It may be dark blond, resembling the "dirty" blond of Summer (but with more golden tones), light golden brown, chestnut, coppery brown, auburn, strawberry, or red. Some Autumns have dark brown or even black-brown hair. These Autumns can tell by the lipstick test that they are indeed an Autumn rather than a Winter! Autumn's eyes are usually brown or green. Autumn blue eyes may have golden or brown flecks in the iris, may look like steel blue from a distance, or may be teal blue or even a bright turquoise. Her skin is ivory, peach, golden beige, or brown, and may look yellow. Like Winter, she rarely has cheek color, and needs blush to "come alive." Some Autumns have ruddy skin with bright red cheeks. Autumns are never olive.

Common combinations for Autumn hair, eye color, and skin tone are:

HAIR	EYES	SKIN
Brown Ivory Charcoal brown Chestnut Coppery brown Red Charcoal black	Beige	Dark brown Yellow beige Swarthy, golden beige Golden brown
Dark golden blond Light golden brown	Dark brown	Ivory Peach Light beige
Brown Auburn	Light golden brown	Ivory Peach
Red Strawberry Dark blond Light auburn	Green with yellow brown flecks Pale, clear green	Ivory Ruddy peach Golden beige
Chestnut Golden brown Red brown Red	Blue with yellow or brown flecks Steel blue Teal Turquoise	Ivory Light beige

Autumn Women: Sophia Loren, Vanessa Redgrave, Meryl Streep, Stephanie Powers, Shirley MacLaine, Sarah Ferguson, Duchess of York.

SPRING

Clothing: The Spring woman shines in clear, warm colors such as light coral, peach, warm pinks, turquoise, salmon, yellow-greens, golden yellow, and orange-red. Blond and redheaded Springs also wear camel, golden brown, peach, and apricot well. Brunette Springs especially love light royal blue, clear red, bright navy, bright golden yellow, periwinkle blue, and medium violet. Blond Springs, unlike blond Summers, cannot wear any muted or dark colors. Dusty mauve will look drab, and dark plum will look harsh and heavy. Brunette Springs look similar to Winters but they are not flattered by blue-based fuchsias or dark blue-reds or burgundy. Redheaded Springs can wear a few Autumn colors, but look better in the lighter, clearer colors of Spring, which give a lift to their faces.

Makeup: Spring glows in clear salmon or warm pink blush, and her favorite lipsticks are clear shades of salmon, coral pink, coral, or peach. Some Springs look better in pink than peach, but the pink must be a yellow-pink rather than a blue-based one. Brunette or redheaded Springs often look wonderful in clear, orange-red lipstick.

Coloring: Springs usually have golden blond, strawberry, light red, or golden brown hair. Some Springs have natural, flaxen blond hair with a bright, clear look to it. A few Springs have medium to dark brown hair with or without red highlights. The majority of Springs have blue or green eyes with yellow flecks, though some have light brown or amber-colored eyes. Spring's skin tone is ivory, peach, golden beige, or brown. A few Springs are ruddy, with pink cheeks. Black Springs are light and golden with a clear, bright look, and Asian Springs have very light, ivory skin.

The most common combinations of Spring hair, eye color, and skin tone are:

HAIR	EYES	SKIN
Flaxen blond	Blue with yellow	Ivory
Golden blond	flecks	Peach
Dark blond with	Green with yellow	Golden beige
golden highlights	flecks	
Strawberry	Green	Ivory
Red	Blue	Peach
Light brown	Light golden	Ivory
Dark blond	brown	Peach
	Amber	Golden beige
Golden brown	Green	Ivory
Reddish brown	Blue	Peach beige
Neutral brown		
Reddish brown	Brown	Ivory (Asian)
Neutral brown		Golden brown

Spring Women: Zsa Zsa Gabor, Christie Brinkley, Sally Struthers, Julie Andrews, Marilyn Monroe, Goldie Hawn, Jane Pauley.

Now that you've chosen one or two seasons that best fit you, it's time to see yourself in makeup colors. Don't worry if you are confused by the descriptions you've just read; the makeup will tell. Seeing is believing.

STEP 2: COMPARING MAKEUP COLORS

Unless you have bags full of cosmetics in a variety of colors, you'll need to go to a store for this test. Wear a white blouse, as it will not clash with any makeup colors you try on. If you wear a fuchsia top and try on a cinnamon lipstick shade, it will clash with the blouse and be hard to judge.

Don't wear any foundation. The one you have at home may be wrong and could be covering up your natural skin tone. You'll determine your proper foundation after you know your season.

I'm going to describe four sets of lipstick and blush colors, one set for each season. You can of course try on all four sets, but that's usually not necessary. Having read the descriptions, you should be able to narrow yourself to two seasons, at most three. After you've determined your season, you'll have the pleasure of investigating all the other makeup colors that will flatter you.

When you go to the store, start with a brand that carries lots of colors. You still may need to use testers from several brands to put together your test colors. I have placed an asterisk (*) next to the best test colors on each makeup palette chart (pages 21, 23, 25, and 27) to further help you find appropriate lipstick and blush colors. In addition, at the back of the book I've included information for more help in determining your season.

For Winter, look for a clear pink blush (or burgundy, if you have very dark skin). Find a lipstick that is a fairly bright pink (or deep pink if your skin is dark). It doesn't have to be screaming, but it shouldn't be too pale. A slightly frosted color is fine.

For Summer, find a soft rose blush. Then, look for a soft rose pink lipstick.

For Autumn, look for a tawny peach blush. Now find a terra cotta or cinnamon lipstick shade.

For Spring, find a clear salmon blush. For lipstick, look for a soft, clear salmon. (Avoid brownish tones.)

As you try on each set, take the time to apply the lipstick carefully. Use a lip pencil if possible (see Chapter 12). You want to give each set of colors a fair look. It's hard to evaluate the attractiveness of a color if it's improperly applied. Crooked lips, or lips with no corners, won't be appealing and will inadvertently influence your opinion of the color.

After you try on the first set, take a good look at yourself in the mirror. It's great if you have a friend come with you for an objective opinion. Or ask the salesperson for her opinion.

Now remove the first set completely. Ask the salesperson for some makeup remover. Powder your cheeks and lips with translucent powder if there is any greasy residue from the remover. Try on the next set. Which is better? If necessary, try on the third and fourth, giving each a proper application and a good look in the mirror.

Which set looks best? When I am testing clients in the stores, I can see a woman's eyes light up when we put on her "right" colors. Sometimes I will put on the wrong colors first, just so she can see the exciting difference in the right ones. She knows that's it!

If you are still having trouble, here are a few of the most common problems:

Blond, blue eyes, between Summer and Spring. Try Summer's soft fuchsia lipstick versus Spring's coral pink.

Brunette, blue or green eyes, between Winter and Spring. Try on Winter's true red or blue-red lipstick versus Spring's orange-red.

Brunette, brown eyes, between Winter and Autumn. Try Winter's true red versus Autumn's orange or brick red.

Redhead, green or blue eyes, between Autumn and Spring. Try Autumn's brownish shade versus Spring's delicate peach.

Brunette, blue eyes, between Summer and Winter. Summer or Winter both wear the same family of colors, but the intensity is different. Try Summer's soft fuchsia versus Winter's bright fuchsia.

Blond, green eyes, between Summer and Autumn. Try Summer's soft pink versus Autumn's tawny peach.

If you still can't decide, you may want to go to a professional color-and-image consultant. (See the back of the book for information.)

Once you have the general set of colors that is most flattering, you know your season. Then you can refine the look and hunt for the perfect color and intensity for your lipstick and blush. And, you can add foundation and eye makeup for a complete look and an absolutely wonderful you.

Isn't it nice to know that with your season settled you now have the power to make perfect choices? No more wasting money on the wrong makeup. You can be wary of promotional or fashion colors—unless they are for you, of course!

Now you know your season, but don't move too fast. Before you buy any makeup, you'll want an organized plan. Cosmetics have become costly, and you want each color you purchase to be truly useful. In the next chapter you'll learn a simple way to have a perfect selection of colors on hand so you'll look wonderful every day.

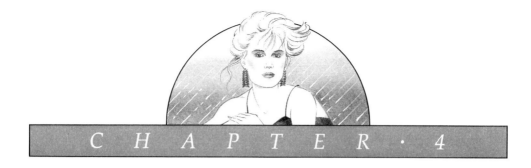

Shopping
for Your
Makeup "Wardrobe"

Now for the fun part—buying your makeup colors! Now that you know your season, it will be easier than ever to shop for makeup. The miracle of Color Me Beautiful is that, because your wardrobe colors all come from one harmonious palette, you can own one blush, one to three lipsticks, and one basic set of eye shadows and they will blend with everything you wear. Even though you have the variety of thirty-six wardrobe colors, plus many of their derivatives, their common warm or cool undertones will be complemented by the similar undertone of your season's makeup palette. Basics are a great way to start, and you'll always look terrific.

Once you get used to wearing your colors and receiving compliments, you may want to acquire some additional makeup colors from your season's palette to match the spectrum of colors in your wardrobe more precisely. It will give you that extra touch of elegance to wear a subtle red-tone blush with a red outfit instead of your basic everyday blush color. Besides, we all get tired of the same thing everyday, and, if you're like me, you'll want some variety.

We'll start by looking at the range of colors in your wardrobe and I'll show you which makeup colors are your most versatile basics. Then, I've included a Makeup Wardrobe Chart to give you some ideas for attractive combinations of wardrobe and makeup colors. I've included an extra, blank chart for each season in the back of the book so you can write in specific names and brands when you shop. You may already own some makeup colors that are just right. If so, write them in. Then you can see what new colors you want to add to your collection. If you feel intimidated by adding extra colors, then stick to the basics. You'll still look great.

When selecting eye shadows, you need to take both your eye color and clothing colors into account. Eye shadow colors will be discussed more fully in Chapter 11, with specific suggestions on how to flatter your eye color. If, later, you see that one of the combinations on the chart is unflattering to your eye color, just cross it off.

Now find the section for your season in the pages that follow. Read the explanation of your season's wardrobe colors and note the exciting ideas for makeup colors. Won't it be fun to have a "wardrobe" of perfect makeup colors, too?

WINInter

WINTER

Lipstick
Look again at the color bar on page 28. The Winter wardrobe has a "blue" end to its spectrum with blue-red, burgundy, fuchsia, and the pinks, as well as a "warmer" end with true red and yellow. For basics, you'll need three colors: pink, true red, and fuchsia lipsticks—they will blend with all the colors in your wardrobe.

To have a perfect lipstick "wardrobe," you can indulge in a range of pink and raspberry shades, plus a fuchsia, two or three reds, and a plum, berry, or burgundy shade. Wear a bluish red lipstick with blue-red clothing. Burgundy clothing is complemented by either burgundy, plum, or raspberry lipstick. Wear fuchsia with fuchsia (most of your other pink lipsticks will not be blue enough), and pink with pink. True red clothing needs true red lip color, and yellow looks best with a geranium red or a pink that is not too blue.

All the other colors in your wardrobe—the neutrals, the blues, and the greens—can be worn with any of the lipstick colors from your palette, whichever are your favorites. If you love pink lips, you can wear pink with green, blue, white, or gray; or, if you are the Snow White type who radiates in red lipstick, you can wear bright red lips with all these wardrobe colors. Black clothing should be worn with a strong color, either red or hot pink or fuchsia, because it is so strong a color itself.

Blush

For perfect harmony, your blush color should match the tone of your lipstick—pink, red, plum, burgundy, or fuchsia—or you can buy one clear pink blush (not too blue) which can blend with pink, red, or fuchsia lip color. If your skin is dark, you might try a burgundy shade for your basic.

Eye Shadow

A basic set of eye shadows would consist of a champagne highlighter, a cool gray contour shade, and either a purple, navy, spruce green, or teal blue shadow, whichever is best for your eye color (see Chapter 11). Your dream eye shadow wardrobe could include the array of colors shown on your makeup palette (see page 21). Your eye shadows can pick up the colors from your clothing, as long as the color looks good with your eye color and is well blended to look subtle. With blue clothing, you can use navy or steel blue shadow; with green clothing, a mint or spruce green; with turquoise, a teal blue or smoky turquoise shadow; with purples and pinks, a purple shadow. You will always use these eye shadows sparingly, mixing and blending them with neutral colors.

Winter Basic Makeup Chart		
Lip Color	**Blush**	**Eye Shadows**
Pink (or Burgundy for dark skins) True Red Fuchsia	Clear Pink (or Burgundy)	Highlighter: Champagne Neutral: Cool Gray Color: Purple or Navy or Spruce Green or Teal Blue

WINTER MAKEUP WARDROBE CHART

Clothing Color	Lipstick	Blush	Eye Shadows	
			Highlighter	Contour Colors
All Pinks Magenta Royal Purple Icy Violet	Pink	Clear Pink	Pale Pink	Gray; Purple
True Red Blue Red	True Red Blue Red	Soft True Red	Champagne	Gray; Navy or Steel Blue or Sapphire Blue or Spruce Green
Fuchsia	Fuchsia	Fuchsia	Pale Pink	Gray; Purple
Bright Burgundy Vivid Cranberry	Plum or Burgundy or Raspberry	Plum or Burgundy	Pale Pink	Gray; Purple or Mauve or Steel Blue or Navy
Lemon Yellow Icy Yellow	Geranium Red Azalea Pink	Soft True Red Clear Pink	Champagne Pale Yellow	Cocoa; Aqua or Teal Blue or Teal Green or Smoky Turquoise or Navy
Bright Periwinkle Blue Royal Blue True Blue Icy Blue	Any	Coordinate with lips	Pale Gray Cool Blue	Gray; Sapphire Blue or Navy or Steel Blue or Purple
Hot Turquoise Chinese Blue Clear Teal Bright Emerald Turquoise Icy Aqua	Pink Fuchsia	Pink Fuchsia	Pale Gray Aqua	Gray; Smoky Turquoise or Teal Blue or Teal Green or Grayed Purple

WINTER MAKEUP WARDROBE CHART (CONTINUED)

Clothing Color	Lipstick	Blush	Eye Shadows	
			Highlighter	Contour Colors
Light True Green True Green Emerald Green Pine Green Icy Green	Any	Coordinate with lips	Champagne Mint	Cocoa; Spruce Green or Purple or Navy
Black White Navy All Grays	Any	Coordinate with lips	Icy Gray	Gray; Any
Black Brown Taupe	Any	Coordinate with lips	Champagne Taupe	Cocoa; Any

SUMMER

Lipstick

Study the color bar on page 29. The Summer wardrobe has a "blue" end to its spectrum with blue-red, burgundy, soft fuchsia, mauve, plum, and the pinks, and a "warmer" end with watermelon red and light lemon yellow. For a basic lipstick collection, you will need three shades: rose pink, soft fuchsia, and watermelon red.

For a complete lipstick wardrobe, you can collect a range of pink and rose shades, as well as a soft fuchsia, a mauve, a plum or wine, and a couple of soft reds. With blue-red clothing wear a bluish red lipstick. With burgundy, choose a wine or plum lipstick. Wear fuchsia with fuchsia; with mauve and plum clothing wear mauve or plum; with pinks wear pink or rose. Watermelon red clothing needs to be paired with a watermelon shade of red lipstick. With yellow, choose watermelon red or a pink lip color that is not too blue. All the other colors in your wardrobe—the neutrals, blues, and greens—can be worn with any of the lip colors on your makeup palette, whichever most flatters you.

Blush
Your blush color ideally should harmonize with your lipstick, so, for a perfect blush collection, you would buy a soft rose or a medium pink, a soft fuchsia, a soft plum or mauve, and a watermelon red. For a basic blush, however, a soft rose (not too blue), will go with pink, red, or fuchsia lip color.

Eye Shadow
A basic set of eye shadows, to go with everything, would consist of a champagne highlighter, a cool gray neutral, and either steel blue, grayed grape, spruce green, or teal blue eye shadow, whichever best complements your eye color (see Chapter 11). Your extended shadow wardrobe can include practically all the colors shown on your makeup palette (see page 23). Your eye shadows can pick up colors from your clothing, as long as the shadow color looks good with your eye color and is well blended to look subtle. With blue clothing you can wear steel blue shadow; with green clothing, mint or spruce green; with aqua and turquoise, an aqua or soft teal; and with pink, plum, or mauve, use a grape shadow. You will always use these eye shadows sparingly, mixing and blending them with neutral shadow colors.

Summer Basic Makeup Chart

Lip Color	Blush	Eye Shadows
Rose Pink	Soft Rose	Highlighter: Champagne
Soft Fuchsia		Neutral: Cool Gray
Watermelon Red		Color: Steel Blue or
		Grape or
		Spruce Green or
		Teal Blue

SUMMER MAKEUP WARDROBE CHART

Clothing Color	Lipstick	Blush	Eye Shadows	
			Highlighter	Contour Colors
All Pinks All Roses Lavender Orchid Medium Violet	Rose Pink	Soft Rose Medium Pink	Pale Pink	Cool Gray; Grape or Lavender or Silvered Mauve
Watermelon Red Blue-Red	Watermelon Red Soft Blue-Red	Watermelon Red	Champagne	Cool Gray; Steel Blue or Spruce Green or Teal Blue
Soft Fuchsia	Soft Fuchsia	Soft Fuchsia	Pale Pink	Cool Gray; Silvered Mauve or Grape or Spruce Green or Steel Blue
Plum All Mauves Raspberry Burgundy/ Maroon	Soft Plum/Berry Mauve Wine	Soft Plum	Pale Pink	Cool Gray; Grape or Spruce Green or Steel Blue or Silvered Mauve
Light Lemon Yellow	Watermelon Red Pink	Watermelon Red Medium Pink	Pale Yellow Champagne	Cocoa; Aqua or Teal Blue or Teal Green or Mint
Powder Blue Sky Blue Cadet Blue Medium Blue Periwinkle Blue	Any	Coordinate with lips	Champagne Pale Gray	Cool Gray; Cool Blue or Steel Blue or Grape
All Aquas Soft Teal	Any	Coordinate with lips	Champagne Aqua	Cocoa or Cool Gray; Aqua or Teal Blue or Grape

SUMMER MAKEUP WARDROBE CHART (CONTINUED)

Clothing Color	Lipstick	Blush	Eye Shadows	
			Highlighter	Contour Colors
All Blue Greens Spruce Green	Any	Coordinate with lips	Champagne Mint	Cocoa; Mint or Spruce Green or Teal Green or Grape
Grayed Navy Grayed Blue Light Blue-Gray Charcoal Blue-Gray	Any	Coordinate with lips	Champagne Pale Gray	Cool Gray; Steel Blue or Grape or Silvered Mauve
Soft White Rose Beige Rose Brown Cocoa	Any	Coordinate with lips	Champagne	Cocoa; Any

AUTUMN

Lipstick

Look again at the color bar on page 30. The Autumn wardrobe ranges from the warm orangish side—with orange-red, orange, pumpkin, terra cotta, and golden yellow—to the "cooler" end—with salmon pink and brown burgundy. For a basic set of lipsticks, you'll need two colors: a cinnamon or terra cotta and a salmon. A great cinnamon will blend with everything in your closet except the salmons and salmon pinks.

To have an ideal lipstick wardrobe, you can indulge in a range of cinnamon, terra cotta, mocha, and peachy colors, a tawny salmon, one or two reds (say, a brick and an orange-red), plus an orange and a mahogany. Your red clothing will look best with a red lipstick; with orange, pumpkin, and yellow clothing, choose an orange shade; with terra cotta and rust, wear a terra cotta lip color. Peach will look most harmonious with a tawny peach lipstick. On the other hand, the pinkish colors in your wardrobe, especially your salmon pink, need to be paired with a salmon lip tone.

All the other colors in your wardrobe—the neutrals, greens, and blues—can be worn with any of the lipstick colors from your palette, whichever are your favorites. Whether you prefer a brownish tone, a peach, or a bright orange-red, you can successfully pair any with your olive or forest green, brown or tan, periwinkle blue, or teal blue clothing. Your warm pewter, because it is grayish, looks best with either a red or mahogany lipstick, rather than a brown one.

Blush

Your blush colors ideally should match your lipstick—peach, chestnut, terra cotta, brick red or salmon. For a basic, buy a tawny peach, which will harmonize reasonably well with all your colors. If your skin is very fair, try a lighter apricot shade.

Eye Shadow

A basic set of eye shadows, to blend with everything, would consist of a champagne highlighter, a bronze contour shadow, and either a teal blue, smoky turquoise, olive green, warm green, or copper eye shadow, whichever is best for your eye color (see Chapter 11). Your dream eye shadow wardrobe could contain all the colors on your Autumn makeup palette (see page 25). Your eye shadows can pick up colors from your clothing, as long as the shadow is attractive with your eye color as well. With blue clothing, you can wear periwinkle; with teal and turquoise, teal shadow; with pumpkin, orange, or brown, choose peach and copper shadow; with greens, wear warm green shadow. Of course you'll want to mix these eye shadows with some of your neutral shades, so they don't look too bright.

Autumn Basic Makeup Chart

Lip Color	Blush	Eye Shadows
Terra Cotta or Cinnamon	Tawny Peach	Highlighter: Champagne
		Neutral: Bronze
Tawny Salmon		Color: Teal Blue or Smoky Turquoise or Olive Green or Warm Green or Copper

---

AUTUMN MAKEUP WARDROBE CHART

| | | | Eye Shadows | |
Clothing Color	Lipstick	Blush	Highlighter	Contour Colors
Orange-Red/ Bittersweet Dark Tomato Red	Orange-Red Brick Red	Brick Red	Champagne	Coffee Brown; Smoky Turquoise or Warm Green or Copper
Brown Burgundy Mahogany	Mahogany Mocha	Mocha	Warm Pink	Coffee Brown; Bronze or Copper
All Peaches/ Apricots	Tawny Peach	Tawny Peach Apricot	Pale Peach	Golden Brown; Teal or Copper
Orange/Pumpkin Terra Cotta Rust	Orange/Pumpkin Terra Cotta	Terra Cotta Chestnut	Champagne Pale Peach	Golden Brown; Copper or Warm Green or Teal Blue or Teal Green
Light Gold/Buff Gold Golden Yellow Mustard	Cinnamon Terra Cotta Tawny Peach Orange-Red	Apricot Tawny Peach	Champagne Pale Golden Yellow	Golden Brown; Teal Blue or Green or Aqua or Bronze
Purple Aubergine/ Eggplant	Orange-Red Orangy Coral Salmon	Brick Red Salmon	Champagne	Bronze; Violet or Warm Green
Salmon Pink Salmon	Tawny Salmon	Salmon	Warm Pink	Putty; Smoky Turquoise or Warm Green
Teal Blue Turquoise Jade Green	Any	Coordinate with lips	Champagne Aqua	Bronze, Teal Blue or Teal Green or Smoky Turquoise

AUTUMN MAKEUP WARDROBE CHART (CONTINUED)

			Eye Shadows	
Clothing Color	Lipstick	Blush	Highlighter	Contour Colors
All Periwinkle Blues	Any	Coordinate with lips	Champagne Beige	Putty; Periwinkle Blue of Violet or Copper
Bright Yellow-Green Forest Green Olive Green Moss Green Grayed Green	Any	Coordinate with lips	Champagne Beige	Bronze; Olive Green or Sage or Warm Green or Copper
Oyster White Warm Beige Khaki/Tan Camel Coffee Brown Dark Brown/ Charcoal Medium Warm Bronze Warm Gray/ Pewter	Mocha Honey Brown Any	Mocha Chestnut Coordinate with lips	Champagne	Coffee Brown; Any
Marine Navy	Any	Coordinate with lips	Champagne	Putty; Any

SPRING

Lipstick

Take another look at the Spring color bar on page 31. Notice that the Spring woman's wardrobe colors range from orange-red, orange, peach, and yellow on the "warm" end, to pinks and violet on the "cooler" end. For basic lipsticks, choose a clear salmon and a poppy red. Because salmon is a cross between orange and pink, it will blend with your peaches, pinks, and even violet, as well as the neutrals, blues, and greens. You'll need poppy to wear with your reds.

To have a complete lipstick wardrobe, you could treat yourself to a range of corals and salmons, a peach, one or two warm pinks, a poppy red, and perhaps a light orange. Orange-red looks best with an orange-red lipstick; orange and peach clothes with peach lipstick; yellow clothing with either peach or coral; and pink and violet clothes with a pink lip color.

The other colors in your wardrobe—the neutrals, greens, and blues—can be paired with any lip color from your palette. Choose your favorite. Warm pink, peach, coral, and even your orange-red lipstick will harmonize equally well with your ivory, navy, yellow or kelly green, periwinkle or aqua clothing.

Blush

An ideal blush wardrobe would contain clear salmon, apricot or peach, a warm pink, and a soft poppy red to match your various lip colors. But for a basic, buy a clear salmon, as it will blend reasonably well with everything.

Eye Shadow

A basic set of eye shadows, to go with everything, would be a champagne highlighter, a golden brown contour shade, and either a teal blue, periwinkle blue, peach, or warm green eye shadow, whichever best complements your eye color (see Chapter 11). Your dream shadow wardrobe can include all the colors on your makeup palette (see page 27). Your eye shadows can pick up colors from your clothing as long as the shadow is flattering to your eye color. With blue clothing you can wear periwinkle blue shadow; with aqua and emerald turquoise, a teal or aqua; with peach, orange, and orange-red, a peach shadow; with green clothes, choose a warm green shadow. You will want to use these eye shadows sparingly, and mix and blend them with neutral shadow colors.

Spring Basic Makeup Chart

Lip Color	Blush	Eye Shadows
Clear Salmon Poppy Red	Clear Salmon	Highlighter: Champagne Neutral: Golden Brown Color: Teal Blue or Periwinkle Blue or Peach or Warm Green

SPRING MAKEUP WARDROBE CHART

Clothing Color	Lipstick	Blush	Eye Shadows	
			Highlighter	Contour Colors
Warm Pastel Pink Coral Pink Clear Bright Warm Pink Medium Violet	Warm Pink Coral Pink	Warm Pink Clear Pink	Warm Pink	Warm Gray; Violet
Clear Salmon	Clear Salmon Salmon Pink	Clear Salmon	Warm Pink	Honey; Teal Blue or Warm Green
Bright Coral	Coral	Clear Salmon Soft Poppy Red	Pale Peach	Golden Brown; Light Copper
All Peaches/ Apricots Light Orange	Peach Apricot Light Orange	Clear Peach Apricot	Pale Peach	Golden Brown; Teal Blue or Warm Green or Sage or Light Copper
Orange-Red Clear Bright Red	Orange-Red Poppy Red	Soft Poppy Red	Pale Peach	Golden Brown; Bronze or Light Copper or Teal Blue

59

SPRING MAKEUP WARDROBE CHART (CONTINUED)

Clothing Color	Lipstick	Blush	Eye Shadows	
			Highlighter	Contour Colors

Buff
Light Clear Gold
Bright Golden
  Yellow
	Peach
	Clear Salmon
	Coral
		Clear Peach
		Clear Salmon
		Poppy Red
			Ivory
			Pale Golden
			  Yellow
				Golden Brown;
				Bronze or Aqua
				or Teal Green or
				Periwinkle Blue

All Yellow-
  Greens
Light True
  Green
Kelly Green
	Any	Coordinate
		with lips
			Champagne
			Pale Golden
			  Yellow
				Golden Brown;
				Warm Green or
				Sage Green or
				Teal Green or
				Bronze

All Periwinkle Blues Light True Blue Medium Blue	Any	Coordinate with lips	Champagne	Honey; Periwinkle Blue or Violet
All Aquas Emerald Turquoise Light Teal Blue	Any	Coordinate with lips	Aqua	Honey; Teal Blue or Teal Green or Aqua

Ivory
Light Warm
  Beige
Camel/Tan
Medium Golden
  Brown
Chocolate Brown
	Any	Coordinate
		with lips
			Ivory
			Champagne
				Honey;
				Any

SPRING MAKEUP WARDROBE CHART (CONTINUED)

Clothing Color	Lipstick	Blush	Eye Shadows	
			Highlighter	Contour Colors
Light Warm Gray Medium Warm Gray Light Clear Navy Clear Bright Navy	Any	Coordinate with lips	Champagne	Warm Gray; Any

SHOPPING FOR MAKEUP

With your Makeup Wardrobe Chart in hand, and your season's printed makeup palette, you are now ready to go shopping!

But even armed with charts and colors, it can still be somewhat overwhelming to look at a tester unit brimming with colorful products. It's hard to know where to begin. Take heart, there is a foolproof *system* to make it easier. Whether you are shopping for foundation or lipstick, the same steps apply. Let's take lipstick. First, separate the lipsticks into warm and cool colors (you'll learn how in later chapters) and pull out the ones that might be for you. Line them up on the counter from light to dark. Start in the middle and try on the medium shade. If it's too dark, put it back in the tester and forget the darker colors. Now try on the next lightest color, then the next lightest, and so on, until you've found the right shade for you. Often the color in the tube, pan, or bottle doesn't look the same on your skin, so trying on the middle shade gives you a starting point. This system also keeps the colors organized, so you don't forget which ones you've already tried on. You'll quickly know whether or not this cosmetic line carries your perfect color. If it does, you've found your color quickly. If not, you needn't agonize. Simply move on to another counter.

This shopping system works especially well for products that are removable from the tester unit. Blushes and eye shadows are usually glued to the unit, so you can't line them up, but you can still use the same principle of starting with the middle shade and then moving lighter or darker.

Often you will not have to do this testing all by yourself. Most salespeople with the major cosmetic lines are familiar with color analysis and are trained beauty advisers, so you will find them quite knowledgeable. Together you can use the "line 'em up, try on the middle" method for finding your perfect shades.

Be sure to check the shade in natural light. Most stores use fluorescent lighting, so you may need to borrow a hand mirror and go to the store entrance or window to evaluate the color. As you try out new products, ask yourself if the color is right (too blue? too yellow?), if the value is flattering (too dark? too light?), and if the color is clear or muted enough for you. You'll soon pinpoint exactly what's right for you!

The beauty adviser can assist you with makeup application. Most of us still love to have personal attention and guidance. If you are not experienced or comfortable with makeup, ask her for help. Tell her *frankly* the look you want. If you feel she is wearing too much makeup for your comfort level, explain that you would like a more natural look. Don't feel intimidated. I assure you the beauty adviser is eager to help you, and a good adviser will always work at your comfort level, not hers.

Shopping for makeup will be more fun than ever now that you know what you're looking for. You won't make costly mistakes, and you can be sure you have invested in good choices that will work for you. Now it's time to bring your makeup home, unwrap all the pretty boxes, and organize your new goodies so they're ready to use at a moment's notice.

ORGANIZING YOUR MAKEUP

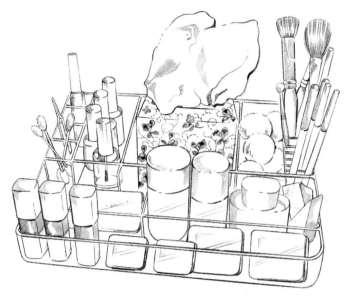

You'll get the most out of your exciting new colors if you buy an attractive plastic organizer and keep your makeup, like your wardrobe, convenient and organized. Place lipsticks in one compartment, blushes in another. Often these organizers have holes for mascara wands and lip and eye pencils. By keeping your makeup orderly and at your fingertips, you'll save time getting dressed in the morning. When I timed myself at putting on my makeup, I noticed that I lost minutes if I had to hunt for a certain eye pencil or lipstick. I can put on all my makeup— foundation, concealer, powder, blush, eyeliner, eye shadow, mascara, and lipstick—in six minutes if I have everything assembled where I need it. An organized "wardrobe" starts the day off smoothly.

Now it's time to acquire the tools you will need to apply your makeup so it looks naturally beautiful—just like you!

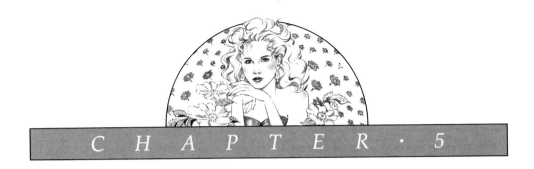

Beauty Tools

Have you ever tried to paint a thin line with a thick brush or with a brush that had hairs sticking out and refused to make a point? I have. My first entrepreneurial venture was a cookie ornament business. I fashioned little "people" out of salt dough, stuck a Christmas hook in their heads, baked them, and painted them. I painted intricate patchwork designs on their dresses and, of course, each had to have a smile, rosy cheeks, and long eyelashes. After painting a number of lopsided smiles and lumpy lashes, I learned the job was impossible without a very thin, pointed sable brush. With the right brush, the job was a cinch.

Before you begin the makeup lesson in Part II, you need the right tools. With good tools, you can control the amount of color you want, blend colors, and correct minor mistakes. Even the finest cosmetics will look streaky applied with poor applicators.

Many women don't buy special brushes because they think they aren't necessary. The tiny applicators inside shadow and blush containers are convenient for touch-ups, but they will not produce as natural and blended a look as full-size quality brushes you purchase separately. After only one practice session, you will use good brushes forever. They will last for years, and you'll never regret the investment.

Do try to buy only natural hair brushes. Natural hair is gentle to your face, lasts longer, maintains its shape, and allows you to control the application. The weight of natural hair also gives a brush the best balance. Pony, goat, sable, camel, and squirrel hairs are commonly used in brushes. Don't panic if your brushes shed a few hairs when new. If they continue to shed after a week or so, however, return them.

Professional-quality brushes and applicators are easy to find in most department stores. Buy a set, if you can, or purchase individual brushes as you can afford them. Packaged as a set, brushes are usually less expensive than buying each separately. Prices for good sets will range roughly from $35 to $65.

Brush sets often come in a roll-type pouch. This is great for travel, but not convenient for daily use. I like to store my brushes upright in a Plexiglas or ceramic cup, something pretty. Make sure your container is not too light, however, or it might fall over from the weight of the brushes. If you travel often, I strongly recommend that you treat yourself to a separate travel-size brush set and keep it permanently packed in your suitcase. One summer vacation when I forgot to pack my brushes I couldn't believe how much harder it was to apply my makeup. It took me twice as long, and the final result was less than satisfactory.

The following brushes would make an ideal, complete set. They are described in the order you would use them. You'll learn more about how to use these brushes in the chapters that follow. If you can't buy a full set just yet, start with a blush brush, powder brush, eye fluff brush, and eye sponge. Add, too, a lip brush, to outline your lips evenly, unless you plan to use a lip pencil.

Under-Eye Brush

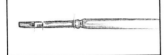

An under-eye brush is like a thin, flat paintbrush, about ¼" wide, and is used to apply concealer or coverstick to dark under-eye circles or lines around the mouth. Also, it's wonderful for highlighting cheek bones. I like to have two of these brushes so I can use the second one to "smudge" eyeliner and soften its effect. Ideally, this brush should be made of natural, resilient sable.

Powder Brush

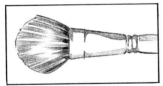

This, the largest brush in your collection, is used to fluff on loose or pressed powder. It should be slightly rounded in shape and very full. Select soft hair such as pony, squirrel, goat, or a combination.

Blush Brush

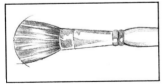

The blush brush is one of your most important tools. Smaller than the powder brush but similar in shape and composition, it's used to apply and blend your blush. This brush ideally should contain some sable, as sable has enough body to help "move" the blush where you want it on your cheek. Correct placement of your blush is key, so please don't skimp on the quality of your blush brush.

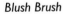

66

Contour Brush

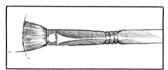

The contour brush looks like a blush brush that has been cut straight across the top. The flat, stubby shape is great for removing excess blush, blending the edges of your blush or eye shadow, or for contouring.

Fan Brush

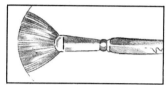

You'll have fun with this thin, soft, fan-shaped brush. Because of the softness of its hair (usually goat), it provides a light application of any powder product. It's ideal for gently removing excess loose powder, for applying iridescent powder at night, or for applying a touch of bright blush when you want the application to be very light. Turned sideways, it can be used to "hollow" your cheekbones with a contour powder.

Eyeliner Brush

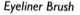
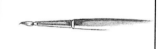

This thin, fine-tipped brush is used wet to apply cake eyeliner or to turn your eye shadow into an eyeliner. Select a brush made of sable so it is resilient, not too soft, and holds its point. If you have blemishes, you can buy a second brush and use it to dot coverstick on the problem spots for extra coverage after foundation has been applied.

Eye Shadow Sponge

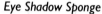
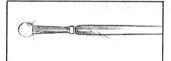

An eye shadow sponge will apply shadow more heavily than the brush, so it is best for applying light to medium colors or any shadows where you want more coverage. A clean sponge is also great for blending stubborn edges, "erasing" mistakes, or—turned sideways—for "smudging" eyeliner to soften its effect. Eye sponges are not expensive, so you'll want to have several. Be sure the applicator is made of cosmetic-grade sponge, which is smooth to the touch. If the sponge looks very porous or is scratchy, don't buy it.

Eye Shadow (Fluff) Brush

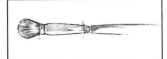

The fluff brush is a miniature version of your blush brush—the same shape and hair. It will give you a light application of eye shadow, and is especially good for dark colors where you don't want too much. You'll also use it for blending.

Eye Contour (Angle) Brush

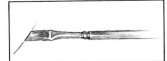

This brush is my favorite because it gives you so much control in the placement of your shadow. Your "angle" brush looks like an under-eye brush that has been sliced diagonally. The shape of the brush is great for fanning shadow along the orbital bone. Here, sable is best, to give the brush substance.

Brow and Lash Brush/Comb

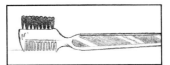

One side of this handy tool looks like a thin, stiff toothbrush, the other like a tiny comb. Use the brush to groom and shape your eyebrows, and use the comb to gently separate your lashes after applying mascara.

Lipstick Brush

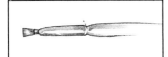

You'll become an expert painter when you use this flat, narrow brush to line your lips and apply lipstick. No lopsided lips for you! Sable is essential for your lipstick brush because it is stiff enough to spread the color and hold its shape for maximum control. I especially like the compact, retractable type because you can carry it in your purse for touch-ups.

Be sure to wash your brushes periodically in mild detergent, then remove excess water with a towel. Don't soak them or the wooden handles will crack. Smooth and shape the hairs on the brushes and lay your damp brushes flat on a towel to dry. They'll dry more quickly if you let the hair extend over your counter so air can circulate. Be careful not to dry your brushes in an upright position, as water may seep into the wooden handles. If you prefer, you can use alcohol, which won't harm natural hair, to clean and sterilize your brushes. Wash at least one eye sponge every day so it will be clean and dry for the next day's use.

In addition to brushes, there are several other tools you'll need. Most are available at any good drugstore.

Cosmetic Sponge

Cosmetic sponges are used to apply and blend foundation. Good sponges are made of dense, cosmetic-grade latex. If you are not sure of the composition, made sure the pores of the sponge are almost invisible and that the sponge feels smooth against your skin. The sponges usually come in triangle or diamond shapes, so the pointed corners can get into the nooks and crannies around your nose and eyes. You may also use your sponge for blending down blush or shadow, if you find you've applied too much. It's a good idea to have several on hand and wash them frequently so you always have a clean, dry one for blending.

Cotton Balls or Pads

These are primarily used for applying skin-care products such as liquid cleansers, tonics, and eye makeup remover, but they can also be used for blending and softening eye shadows and blush. If you have sensitive skin, make sure you buy real cotton rather than synthetic balls and pads. Synthetic fibers can be abrasive and are also less absorbent than cotton.

Cotton Swabs

You can use swabs to "smudge" and blend eyeliners and shadows, or to remove mascara mistakes.

Tissues

Tissues are handy for wiping up spills or cleaning brushes, but use them sparingly on your skin. Paper is made of wood fiber, and the slightly rough texture can irritate sensitive skin.

Tweezers

Tweezers are for plucking stray hairs from your eyebrows. You have a wide selection of styles from which to choose, but my favorite type resembles a pair of scissors.

Eyelash Curler

This tool requires great care and a steady hand. (You don't want to break off or pull out your lashes.) It works on a clamp-pressure principle, putting a crimp in your lashes so they curl upward. Rinse the rubber pad after every use and have an extra one available if you use the curler often. Curl your lashes first, then apply mascara.

Sharpener

If you use lip or eye pencils, a sharpener is an absolute must. Many pencil products come with a sharpener, but if not, you can use the type sold with school supplies. If you find your soft lip pencils or smudgeliners breaking in the sharpener, try popping them into the freezer for a few minutes before sharpening.

Mirrors and Lights

If you don't have good lighting in your makeup area, you may want to purchase a mirror with lights. Many have adjustable light settings that duplicate the lights in an office, daytime, evening, or home setting. No one stays in one place all day, so set your mirror on the brightest setting so you can see what you're doing. Good lighting that doesn't cast a shadow is more important than the color of the light (unless you are going out for dinner and want to know how you'll look in an evening setting). A magnifying mirror is handy when you are plucking your eyebrows or if you have difficulty seeing in a normal mirror.

Shopping List
Here is a list of all your beauty tools. Check off the items you already have and use the list as your shopping guide.

_____ Under-Eye Brush

_____ Powder Brush

_____ Blush Brush

_____ Contour Brush

_____ Fan Brush

_____ Eyeliner Brush

_____ Eye Shadow Sponges (two)

_____ Eye Shadow (Fluff) Brush

_____ Eye Contour (Angle) Brush

_____ Brow and Lash Brush/Comb

_____ Lipstick Brush (two—one for purse)

_____ Brush Cup

_____ Cosmetic Sponges (several)

_____ Cotton Balls or Pads

_____ Cotton Swabs

_____ Tissues

_____ Tweezers

_____ Eyelash Curler

_____ Sharpener

_____ Magnifying Mirror and Lights

Now you have everything you need to become your own makeup artist. You're almost ready to begin your adventure into the Makeup Lessons. But first, if you're going to be an artist, you need to prepare your canvas. . . .

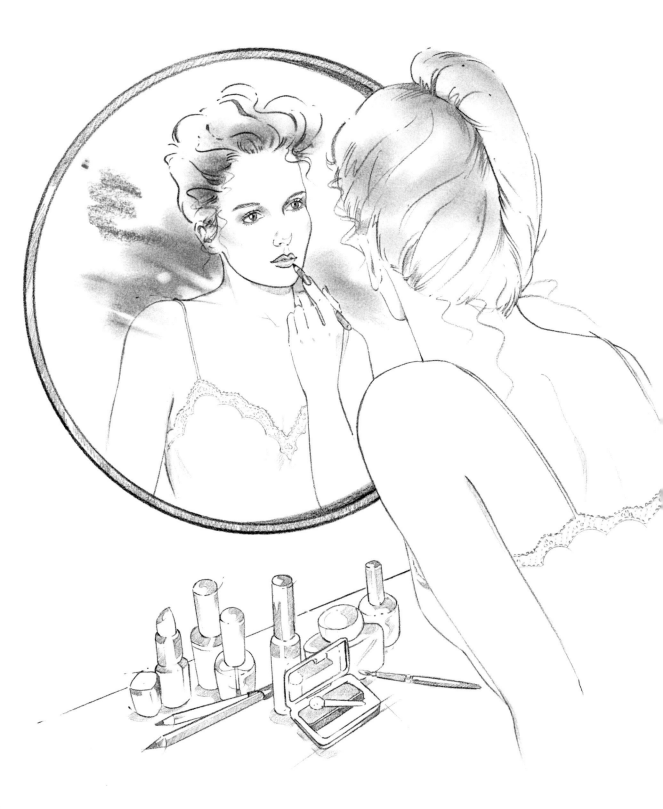

Part II

The Makeup
Lesson

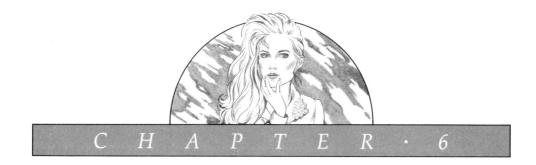

CHAPTER 6

Skin Care

You've found your season, you know your colors, you've assembled your beauty tools—but wait! Before you put even a dab of makeup on your face, you *must* have skin that's squeaky clean and well cared for. If you skimp on skin care, nothing that comes after will look its best.

When I do makeovers on my promotional tours, I frequently find women whose skin is parched and dry, even rough. When I ask what skin care products they use, I often hear, "Well, I wash my face with whatever soap is in the shower, and sometimes throw on a little moisturizer." Such skin, abused by harsh body soap and starving for moisture, will slurp up the foundation, leaving it thick and cakey-looking. Not only will poor skin care wrinkle your skin prematurely, but you also will be depriving yourself of one of your potentially greatest assets—beautiful skin.

I can understand a woman's reluctance to move from soap and water into a modern skin-care routine. With so many new products on the market, we all have been confused about which to buy and how to use them. I assure you, however, that the benefits are well worth the effort of learning how to pamper your skin. All our grandmothers had was Ivory soap and cold cream to combat the aging process, but we have the benefit of recent dramatic breakthroughs in skin-care research and products. Now there are special new ingredients—especially enzymes and vitamins—that help retard wrinkling and keep our skin looking smooth and supple.

You are probably wondering if you have *time* for an elaborate skin-care routine. Don't panic. I promise you, it takes longer for me to describe the routine and the products than it will for you to use them.

The general principles of skin care show good common sense. First, you thoroughly clean your skin, occasionally using a scrub to remove dead skin cells. (The accumulation of those dead cells is what causes rough, scaly skin.) Then, you soften and tone your skin with a toner or astringent, which also helps your skin maintain its elasticity. Next—and this is the new part—you *nourish* the cells while they are growing so they will arrive at the surface as round and plump as possible (the only part of our bodies we like to have plump!). Then you seal in your skin's moisture with a moisturizer. And, last, you lubricate your eye area. The whole routine takes five minutes or less. Time yourself. You'll see.

Every couple of weeks or so, you may also want to bleach or remove excess facial hair, if you have any. Some women need to pluck and shape their eyebrows, or bleach or wax off a mustache. Then your skin will be smooth, free of fuzz, and ready for makeup. You'll love the results.

DETERMINING YOUR SKIN TYPE

Before I explain your routine, let's take a minute to identify your type of skin, since this will affect your skin-care regimen. Filling in the questionnaire that follows, you'll learn whether your skin is dry, normal, oily, or a combination. Women with combination skin have normal cheeks but an oily forehead, nose, and chin (commonly called the T-zone).

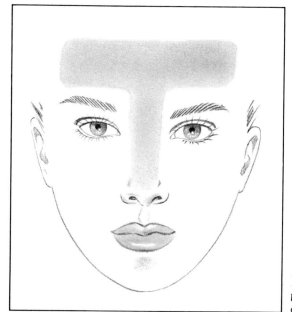

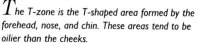
*T*he T-zone is the T-shaped area formed by the forehead, nose, and chin. These areas tend to be oilier than the cheeks.

In the chart on the next page, circle the answers that apply to your skin and then add up your responses in each column. The column that contains the most circles determines your basic skin type. If your circles are split fairly evenly between two columns, place yourself in the oilier category. It's better to err on the side of a regimen that is less rich, since overly rich products can cause breakouts. You can always switch to richer products if you need them.

You may need to reassess your skin type from time to time. Many factors—a personal crisis, stress, getting married or divorced, pregnancy, taking on a new job, taking certain medications, or simply getting older—can affect your skin. Often a change in climate or environment will affect your skin's balance. During hot, humid weather your skin may become so oily that you'll need little or no moisturizer. During the winter, cold weather, heated houses, and dry air can parch even normal and combination skins. Be sensitive to how your skin looks and

QUESTION	DRY	NORMAL/ COMBINATION	OILY
Do you break out?	Rarely	Occasionally	Frequently
Do you have blackheads?	Few or none	Some in T-zone	Problem
What do your pores look like?	Nearly invisible	Visible in T-zone	Enlarged
After washing with soap, how does your skin look and feel in one hour, without a moisturizer?	Dry and tight	Slightly tight for the first half hour, comfortable or with some oil in T-zone by the end of an hour	Oily in half an hour; shiny nose and forehead in one hour
What is your coloring?	Very fair; fair	Fair to medium	Olive to dark
Do you have facial lines?	Some around eyes, lips, forehead	A few around eyes	None or very few
How do you respond to the sun?	Burn easily	Usually burn first, then tan gradually	Rarely burn, tan easily

feels. Adjust your regimen to use more, or less, of any product, depending on your skin's needs. If, for example, your skin is on the borderline between normal and oily, you may want to skip your moisturizer for several days during oily bouts. Or, your skin may need products for dry skin during the wintertime, but those for normal skin during the summer months.

Don't forget that what you put into your body affects your skin. Eat plenty of fruits and vegetables—the high-water-content foods—and drink pure water to hydrate your skin from the inside. Avoid fats, caffeine, and cigarettes. Fats are indigestible, caffeine overstimulates the adrenal glands, and both can cause breakouts and increased oil production. Cigarettes constrict the blood vessels, limiting the oxygen supply to the skin (look at the wrinkles around the eyes of a heavy smoker). Get sleep so your skin can rest. Get aerobic exercise so your whole body gets the benefit of increased circulation.

Your skin is the largest organ in your body! It reflects the condition of your health and your spirit. Take good care of it.

STEPS TO GOOD SKIN CARE

With your skin type in mind, you're ready to choose the products that will enhance your lovely skin, and to master your skin-care program so it will be as natural as brushing your teeth. There are five basic categories of skin-care products: *cleansers, toners, nourishers* (which include cell-renewal formulas), *moisturizers,* and *special eye-area lubricants.* As we go through the five steps of a basic skin-care regimen, we'll look at each product and the role it will play in your personal routine. You'll find specific information for your skin type in the skin-care charts on pages 86 to 88.

Shopping for skin-care products will be easy because each cosmetics company designs formulas for the different skin types. I strongly suggest that you purchase the same brand for all your skin-care needs. The products within each line are designed to work together; if you buy cleanser from one company, nourisher from another, and moisturizer from a third, you risk getting too much of one ingredient or not enough of another.

STEP 1: CLEANSING

The cornerstone of your skin-care program is cleansing—getting your face deep-down clean but without stripping it of its essential oils. You'll need to buy a special facial cleanser and use it twice a day, just as you brush your teeth. (You can take it into the shower, if you like. See—you don't have to change all your habits!) Cleansers come in a range of forms—liquids, gels, creams, oils, and bars (facial soaps).

Gently massage your cleanser in an upward and circular motion to thoroughly remove dirt from under the downy facial hairs and the surface of the pores. Use your fingertips, a soft washcloth, or a cosmetics brush (my favorite!). Turn a boring task into a treat by giving your face a minimassage each time you cleanse.

SUPERCLEANSING
Your daily cleansing will leave your skin clean and soft, but occasionally you will want to supplement it with a supercleanser—a special scrub or mask designed to remove dead skin cells and to deep-clean your pores. Dead cells, if allowed to remain, can cause roughness and can also lead to whiteheads or bumpiness. If you use a cellular renewal product, which generates new cell growth quickly, your supercleansers are especially important.

Scrubs are mildly abrasive, and are primarily for removing dead skin; masks help cleanse the pores. Both invigorate and stimulate the skin. You can use either scrub or mask, or both—with scrub first followed by your mask. You will *love* the way your skin feels. As with other skin-care products, scrubs and masks come in formulas especially for your skin type, so be sure to check the labels.

Scrubs These often contain cleansing grains. Choose one with small, smooth grains such as confectionary-grade nuts, cornmeal, or oatmeal. Avoid those that contain nut shells or kernels, as these are rough and can abrade the skin.

If your scrub comes in a tube, squeeze out a teaspoonful onto the palm of your hand. If your scrub comes in a jar, use a spatula or small spoon. (It's best not to put your finger in the jar, as you risk depositing bacteria.) With your fingertips, massage the scrub into your skin for several minutes in an upward, circular motion on your face and neck, avoiding your eye area. Rinse thoroughly with warm water. Mmmmm! What smooth skin you have!

Masks Some masks contain mud and clay-based compounds that absorb excess oils and draw out dirt and impurities. These mud masks are meant for normal and oily skin types and should not be used by women with dry skin.

Special moisturizing masks, usually made with honey, cleanse and mildly stimulate the skin and also attract moisture from the air, helping to plump up the cells on the surface of your skin. Although these masks are primarily for dry skin, any skin type can benefit from a moisturizing mask from time to time, especially when the weather is cold and dry, or if skin has been exposed to excessive wind or sun.

Apply your mask in a thin, even layer, avoiding your eye area. If you use a mud mask, allow it to dry and become "stiff." The hydrating masks do not stiffen. Follow the directions on the package, and be careful not to overdo—more time is *not* better, especially with a mud mask. Now, gently rinse off your mask with warm water and pat your face dry with a clean, soft towel.

STEP 2: TONING

After cleansing—and supercleansing—you apply your toner. Your toner (which may be called a "freshner" "astringent," "rinse," or even "skin softener") will remove any last traces of cleanser and excess oil, temporarily tighten your skin's surface, and return your skin to its normal pH level, thus protecting it from bacteria. (Cleansing removes the protective "acid mantle" from your skin, and it takes your body about twenty minutes to restore it by itself.) Many toners also have ingredients to soften the skin, making it ready to receive the nourishers or moisturizers to follow.

Toners are applied with a cotton ball or pad, again in an upward direction, from the base of your throat to your hairline. Don't rub hard; it doesn't help the toner clean any better and can harm your skin. Avoid the delicate eye area, as any toner can be drying. Use your toner twice a day, following your regular cleansing or supercleansing with a scrub or mask. Toner leaves your face feeling tingling and refreshed.

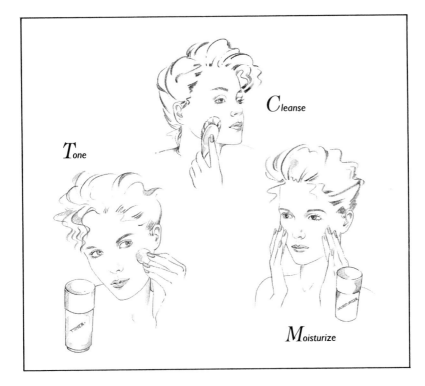

STEP 3: NOURISHING

The next step toward beautiful skin is *nourishing*, an amazing new concept that has emerged from skin-care research over the past five or six years. All skin types can benefit from nourishers, which work underneath the skin's surface, feeding the internal layer of growing cells so they will mature plump and healthy. Nourishers include cell-renewal products as well as wrinkle creams and "anti-aging" lotions, all of which aim to combat the wrinkling process before it begins. A woman will usually begin using a nourisher in her late twenties, when her cell growth begins to slow down.

Nourishers are applied sparingly. They are usually thin, nongreasy, and meant to be followed by moisturizer. Most of the cell-renewal products come in a bottle with an eye dropper. You simply squeeze three to five drops on your fingertips and feather them on to your face. For the creams, you dab just a little on your fingertips and again feather onto your face. Allow these products to dry for a minute or two before applying moisturizer. Use nourisher twice a day, following your toner.

STEP 4: MOISTURIZING

Now it's time to lubricate and protect the *surface* of your skin. Moisturizers will not "erase" wrinkles and cannot repair damaged or aging skin. They do, however, contain humectants, substances that attract water from the air and hold it to the surface of the skin, which helps plump the surface cells. In addition, they contain sealers to hold in the skin's own moisture (water) and to prevent impurities from entering the pores.

A word of caution: Never use petroleum jelly as a moisturizer—it suffocates the skin, causing the pores to enlarge (permanently) in the skin's desperate effort to breathe. Also avoid moisturizers with mineral oil as it too prevents the skin from breathing. Your skin needs oxygen as much as you do!

Whatever your skin type, keep in mind that your skin's moisture needs will vary. The way your skin feels is the best guide. If your skin starts to feel taut, itchy, or rough, it may be time for you to try a richer formula. On the other hand, if you are getting shiny spots on your forehead and nose, or if your skin starts to break out, switch to a lighter product. Everyone needs to use moisturizer on the neck because, without oil glands, it is one of the first areas of our body to show aging.

Apply a thin coat of moisturizer from the base of your throat to your hairline, or in drier areas only, using gentle, upward strokes. Avoid your eye area, as the humectants in the moisturizers can puff up the skin and can cause swelling around your eyes. This will actually stretch the skin and cause wrinkles. Apply just enough moisturizer to do the job. Once again, more is not better; the excess will simply pool on the surface of your skin.

STEP 5: LUBRICATING YOUR EYE AREA

Your skin regime so far has avoided the area around your eyes. Why? Because the skin in your eye area is devoid of oil glands, is extra-thin and delicate, is prone to wrinkling, and needs special care. You need eye cream—different from your moisturizer—with special ingredients and no humectants.

Before lubricating your eye area, you need to thoroughly remove your eye make-up. It's important to remove your eye makeup every night with utmost care. Always use special eye makeup remover, rather than soap, which is too drying. Eye makeup remover comes in liquid, gel, and cream forms and in oily and non-oily formulas. I prefer the non-oily kind for regular use because it's not greasy and if you accidentally get some in your eye, it won't blur your vision. Also, it's wonderfully handy to have around for repairing eye makeup mistakes. A cotton swab dipped in eye makeup remover can erase unwanted dots of mascara or eye shadow like magic without ruining the rest of your makeup. If you are removing waterproof mascara, you'll need to purchase one of the oily formulas specifically for waterproof mascara. Any eye makeup remover should not sting. If it does, it undoubtedly contains an ingredient to which you are sensitive, so switch to another brand.

To use eye makeup remover, dab a small amount on a cotton ball, wipe downward on your upper lid, and then across under your lower lashes, from the outside corner in. Don't saturate the cotton, or you can wash makeup into your eyes.

After you've completely removed your eye makeup, you're ready to lubricate the skin around your eyes. Eye creams vary from heavy ointments to lightweight creams and gels, and are formulated for all skin types. The ointments are better for night because they are a bit tacky, while the lighter weight products can be worn even under makeup. Look for a formula containing vitamin E, an excellent natural lubricant.

To apply eye cream, use your ring finger—it's the weakest—so you won't stretch or pull your skin. Gently pat a tiny amount of cream along your orbital bone (the one that encircles your eye). Don't apply the cream too close to your lashes, as the warmth of your body can make it melt and spread into your eye. Use eye cream twice a day, following moisturizer.

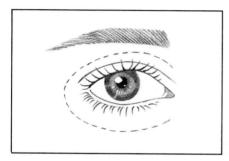

*T*he orbital bone is the bone that surrounds your eye.

If your eyes are red and puffy from allergies, too much sleep, or even from crying, you also might want to try one of the wonderful new eye gels designed specifically to combat puffiness. These gels reduce the accumulation of water under and around the eyes and leave them feeling cool and refreshed. You simply pat the gel on the puffy area before you apply eye cream.

Following are skin-care regimen charts, summarizing the steps for each skin type. I've included the regimens again at the back of the book on a chart you can cut out. I like to keep the regimens for all three types taped to the inside of my medicine cabinet. Then, if I need to adjust my routine for any reason, I have all the steps handy for easy reference. You might also want to consider lining up your products in order in your medicine cabinet or wherever you will store them, and *numbering* them with stickers or a marking pen. I found that when I first added nourisher and scrub to my regimen, I spent a fair amount of time reading labels, trying to remember what came after what. After a few days of practice, you'll know your routine by heart. And, in a few short weeks, you'll really see a difference in your beautiful skin!

SKIN-CARE REGIMEN FOR DRY SKIN

STEP 1: CLEANSING

Choose a cream, liquid, or oily cleanser. These can be rinsed off with warm water or, if your skin is extremely dry, just wiped off with a soft, clean cloth. If you prefer a soap, choose one that is superfatted and made with emollients and moisturizers specifically for dry skin.

Supercleansing. Alternate using a gentle scrub or a honey mask formulated for dry skin once a week after using your regular cleanser. It's OK to use both, on occasion, with mask following scrub, as long as your skin is not extremely sensitive. Caution: Mud masks are not appropriate for dry skin.

STEP 2: TONING

Follow cleansing/supercleansing with toning. You need a toner with no alcohol, since alcohol is too harsh for your skin. Look for a toner that includes witch hazel, the nondrying ingredient most often substituted for alcohol that also helps tighten the surface of the skin. If your skin is *very* dry, you may want to use toner only once a day.

STEP 3: NOURISHING

Apply a few drops of a cell-renewal product or one of the "anti-aging" creams specifically labeled "nourisher," not moisturizer.

STEP 4: MOISTURIZING

Choose a rich moisturizer for daytime and night cream for night. During the winter, you may even want to use your night cream in the daytime if your skin feels rough or chapped. Don't forget to moisturize your neck.

STEP 5: LUBRICATING YOUR EYE AREA

Use an eye cream morning and night.

A.M.	P.M.
Cleanser	Eye makeup remover
Toner	Cleanser
Nourisher	Toner
Rich moisturizer	Nourisher
Eye cream	Night cream
	Eye cream

SKIN-CARE REGIMEN FOR NORMAL OR COMBINATION SKIN

STEP 1: CLEANSING

Try a liquid cleanser or facial bar soap, whichever you prefer. Liquid cleansers for normal skin must be rinsed off, as they usually contain a mild facial detergent, an ingredient not found in products for dry skin.

Supercleansing. Use a scrub or mask (or both) formulated for normal or combination skin once a week after using your regular cleanser.

STEP 2: TONING

Try a nonalcohol toner in the wintertime or in drier climates when your skin might tend to become a bit dry or sensitive. In warmer, more humid climates, you can use an astringent with a small amount of alcohol.

STEP 3: NOURISHING

Apply a few drops of cell-renewal product or other skin-nourishing product of your choice. You may want to apply this product only at night, especially if you are oily in the T-zone.

STEP 4: MOISTURIZING

Choose a lightweight moisturizer for the summer and a slightly richer one for the winter. In the wintertime you may also want to use a night cream. If you have combination skin, use moisturizer only on the cheeks and necks, leaving the oily T-zone alone. After five minutes, if your skin feels at all tacky, pat a cotton ball slightly dampened with toner over your face to remove excess moisturizer that wasn't absorbed.

STEP 5: LUBRICATING YOUR EYE AREA

Use eye cream morning and night.

A.M.	P.M.
Cleanser or beauty bar	Eye makeup remover
Toner/Astringent	Cleanser or beauty bar
(Nourisher)	Toner/Astringent
Moisturizer	(Nourisher)
Eye cream	Moisturizer or Night Cream
	Eye cream

SKIN-CARE REGIMEN FOR OILY SKIN

STEP 1: CLEANSING

Most women with oily skin prefer the feel of a facial soap. Try an oatmeal soap, for its mild abrasiveness will remove dead cells that tend to cling to oily skin. You might also want to help remove excess oil by filling your sink with hot water and rinsing your face with twenty splashes to steam open your pores. Be careful not to wash your face too often in an effort to rid it of oil. Twice a day is enough. If stripped of all its oils, your clever skin will pump overtime and you'll be oilier than ever.

Supercleansing. Use a scrub formulated for oily skin twice a week and a mask once a week after using your regular cleanser.

STEP 2: TONING

Select an astringent with alcohol listed as one of the first five ingredients. Look for products with boric acid, which is antibacterial and helps absorb oil.

STEP 3: NOURISHING

Use a lightweight nourishing product, preferably one with little or no oil. Usually the cell-renewal liquids (the ones that come with the eyedropper) are best for oily skins. Use only at night if your skin is very oily.

STEP 4: MOISTURIZING

You may not need moisturizer for your face—your skin's own oil is often enough—but do moisturize your neck. During the dry winter months, you may want to use a lightweight moisturizer on your cheeks. Some companies produce moisturizers specifically formulated for oily skin—effective in keeping the surface of the skin smooth without adding unwanted oil. If your skin breaks out, it's best to skip all moisturizer (except on your neck). Your skin will dry out as you age so you will eventually need to use moisturizer. If moisturizer seems tacky five minutes after you have applied it, pat a cotton ball slightly dampened with astringent over your face to remove what wasn't absorbed.

STEP 5: LUBRICATING YOUR EYE AREA

Use eye cream morning and night.

A.M.		P.M.	
Cleansing bar	Moisturizer on neck	Eye makeup	Moisturizer on
Astringent	or as needed	remover	neck or as
(Nourisher)	(Astringent/Toner)	Cleansing bar	needed
	Eye Cream	Astringent	(Astringent/Toner)
		Nourisher	Eye Cream

FACIAL HAIR

Upper Lip

Some of us are "blessed" with a fuzzy mustache on our upper lip. Take heart, however, as it's easy to bleach it so the hairs will become blond and barely noticeable. There are several excellent products easily obtained in a drugstore, designed especially for facial hair. If your mustache is thick, I recommend having it removed. The hairs will interfere with the application of your lipstick and ruin your lovely lipline. One option is to wax it off, which is temporary and must be repeated every so often. Most beauty salons offer waxing as a service, or you can buy a waxing kit in the drugstore and do it yourself. If you prefer, you can have hair permanently removed by means of electrolysis or the Depilatron procedure. Check your phone book to locate these services.

Eyebrows

You may also want to shape your eyebrows by plucking hairs that stray too far down on your orbital bone. Your eye shadow won't look as attractive if you have to apply it on top of stray hairs, plus a nice, arched brow will open and lift your eyes. Go easy here, however. Thin or thick eyebrows may or may not be the fashion, but whatever the vogue, never overpluck your brows. Plucked eyebrows often *will not* grow back. A natural look, neither too thin nor too thick, is timeless and always flattering.

Because your eyebrows frame your eyes, it's important that the length of your brow be in proportion to your eye. The illustration shows you how to determine the proper length.

First place a pencil or long-handled brush from the outer edge of your nose to your tear duct. Then place it from your nose to the crease at the outer edge of your eye. Pluck any stray hairs that extend beyond these boundaries. Then pluck the stray hairs underneath your brows. Create a gentle arch, following the shape of your eyes, with the peak at the outside of your pupil. Place your pencil or brush handle from your nose to your pupil to find where the peak should be.

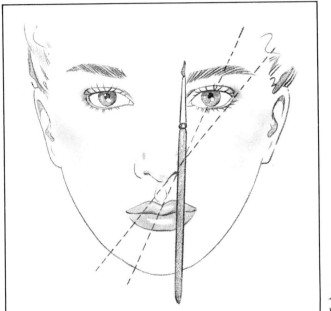

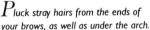
*P*luck stray hairs from the ends of
your brows, as well as under the arch.

...AND THE REST OF YOU

Don't neglect the rest of your body, either. Always keep legs and underarms free of stubbly hair. Follow every bath or shower with lotion on legs, arms, hands, and elbows, perhaps using a favorite scented lotion, to prevent itchy dryness. And, every now and then, indulge in a "Day of Beauty." A day of relaxation and special attention to your needs will enhance your inner beauty, as well as your skin.

By the way, your husband or your boyfriend can use the same products you do. Men's skin care lines are packaged differently, but the products are the same. His skin needs tender loving care just as much as yours. Why not have a facial night together once a month or so—a chance to indulge, and turn off the cares of the world.

A DAY OF BEAUTY

A Day of Beauty is a lovely way to make you feel as special as you are. Just follow these easy steps:

1. Start by washing your hair, using your favorite shampoo.

2. Then fill the tub with clean, comfortably warm water and the additives of your choice—a nice bubble bath or a scented bath oil to soften your skin.

3. While the bath is running, towel dry your hair and apply a generous amount of deep conditioner. Don't rinse your hair yet, just cover it with a shower cap and then wrap it in a towel to let your conditioner penetrate slowly.

4. Now slip into the tub. Soak for a full five or ten minutes, banishing all your tension and worries. Then:

• Work a pumice stone over your feet, heels, and elbows to smooth away rough calluses.

• Lather up a loofa sponge with your most luxurious soap and gently stroke it upward, from your toes to your shoulders, concentrating on rough spots.

5. Rinse yourself off, then step out of the tub and blot yourself dry with a towel.

6. Slather yourself with a rich body lotion, maybe in your favorite fragrance, massaging it especially well into the dry areas of your body.

7. Wrap up in your warm terry cloth robe.

8. Now that your face is nicely steamed from your bath, cleanse it well, massaging it lightly with your fingertips to smooth away muscle tension. Rinse, and give your face a once over with your scrub to leave it glowing and super smooth.

9. Now treat yourself to a mask, according to your skin type. Apply the mask in your bathroom and then, while the mask works, lie down on your bed, feet up, eyes closed, muscles relaxed, mind serene—perhaps with your favorite music in the background.

10. Now, return to the bathroom to rinse the mask off with warm water, and rinse the conditioner out of your hair. You'll want to keep your pampered body dry, so rinse your hair in the sink—first with warm water, then cool. Towel dry your hair and comb it out gently. Give it a chance to dry free in the air, a rest from the blow dryer.

11. Finish your "facial" with toner, nourisher, moisturizer (if needed), and eye cream. Pat eye cream onto your lips as well for an extra soothing touch.

12. If you can keep the world at bay a little longer, curl up with a hot cup of herb tea and a great book, and enjoy.

INGREDIENTS AND SENSITIVITIES

Most of today's skin-care products are a combination of advanced scientific technology and select herbs and botanicals with a proven history of gentle soothing and healing. Many of our great-grandmothers' home remedies really did work!

Skin-care products typically contain *emollients* (mostly oils and silicones to seal in moisture and soften the skin), *humectants* (to add more moisture), *protectants* (to heal and soothe), *emulsifiers* (to make the ingredients work together), *preservatives* and *antioxidants* (so the product won't spoil), as well as the herb and plant extracts and the newer "special" ingredients.

In selecting your skin-care products, look for ingredients such as hyaluronic acid (to add moisture), collagen amino acids (protein to nourish the growing cells), hydrolized elastin (to add moisture and enhance elasticity), retinol (vitamin A), and vitamin E (an emollient and an antioxidant, which supposedly helps prevent aging through cellular breakdown). Products that are in amino acid form have molecules that are small enough to penetrate the surface layer of your skin and help those baby cells that are still growing. Products that say "soluble" have heavier molecules, and work only on the surface of the skin.

Some natural ingredients that are especially beneficial are sesame, sweet almond, and wheat germ oils (emollients), lanolin (a waxy emollient and an excellent skin softener), allantoin (to protect, heal, soothe, and inhibit allergic reaction), the queen bee's "royal jelly" (vitamin B), as well as extracts of aloe vera, apricot kernel, birch leaf, chamomile, clover blossom, coltsfoot, rosemary, and sage (to either soften, soothe, or stimulate the skin).

Don't panic if your skin breaks out a bit after you begin a new skin-care regimen, especially if you hadn't been caring for it beforehand. Your new cleansing regimen will open your pores and pull dirt and hardened oils to the surface, possibly causing temporary blemishes. If you are still having problems after two or three weeks, you may be using a product that is too rich, or you may be allergic.

Allergies usually cause redness and irritation rather than blemishes. Before throwing out your entire regimen, first check for other culprits. Have you begun or stopped using any medication? Changed your shampoo, your mousse, or your laundry detergent? Used a new nail polish, hand cream, or perfume? Even a change in weather and the arrival of pollens or molds can suddenly make you seem "allergic" to a product.

Then, too, make sure that you are following directions carefully. If a cleanser says "rinse thoroughly," not doing so could leave detergent on the skin and result in itching.

If you do have an allergic reaction to a product, you'll have to read labels and be a detective to hunt down the offending ingredient. There is no such thing as a nonallergenic product. Even hypoallergenic lines can contain ingredients that cause reactions in some people. Buying a product that says "allergy tested" does mean, however, that the product does not contain commonly irritating ingredients.

Some ingredients that can irritate sensitive skin are sodium laurel sulfate (a detergent), fragrances, preservatives, and some oils. Almond oil, lanolin, and vitamin E, in spite of their wonderful properties as emollients, can irritate certain very sensitive skins. Mineral oil should be avoided in moisturizers, but does an excellent job in cleansers that are washed off. If you have acne-prone skin, avoid products in which oil is one of the first few ingredients, and do consult a dermatologist. Treatment for acne has improved dramatically over the last five years.

Good skin care takes only minutes a day, and it can make such a dramatic difference! Your face is the image you present to the world. It's worth a little bit of time and effort to keep your skin healthy and glowing.

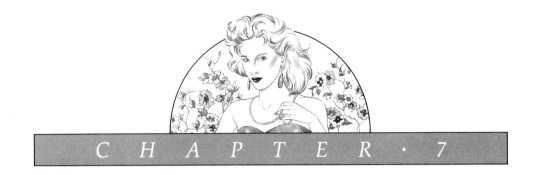

Foundation

Just as an artist prepares a canvas with a special, neutral wash to even out its surface color and imperfections, your face needs foundation to smooth its texture and to even out its tone.

My first experience wearing foundation was appearing in my high school play, when the director had us put on theatrical pancake makeup. It was so greasy and heavy that my face felt dirty, and after that experience I shied away from foundation for years. I couldn't believe the difference when I tried it again. Modern foundation products are sheer, light, and comfortable. You won't even *feel* a foundation if the product is right for you.

Some women avoid foundation because they think it will clog their pores. Ironically, these same women will apply blush and eye shadows directly on their skin, a practice that is far more likely to clog pores. Foundation actually protects your skin (and your pores) from dirt and pollutants and helps reduce moisture loss from the sun and the wind.

CHOOSING THE RIGHT COLOR

The key to a natural look is choosing the right color foundation, one that harmonizes with your skin tone. Women often tell me that finding a foundation to match their skin is a frustrating job. How well I remember "matching" my olive skin, only to turn orange an hour later! Don't despair. Finding the perfect color is going to be easier now that you know your season.

I recommend shopping for foundation in a department store that supplies testers, rather than in a drugstore, where all the packages are sealed. Foundation in the bottle usually looks darker than it does on skin, so you really have to try it on to judge.

To find the perfect foundation, you need to identify the range of shades appropriate to your season. If you are a Winter or a Summer, you want to find *cool* or rose-based shades. Usually colors labeled *rose, sand, rachel, mahogany,* or *neutral* are cool. Autumns and Springs should look for *warm* or yellow-based shades. These often are called *porcelain, ivory, peach, golden, bronze,* or *natural.* If you find colors with nondescriptive names such as Beige Delight, ask the salesperson if she knows which colors in her line are rose-based or yellow-based.

If she doesn't know, you will have to judge by eye. Some colors will be obviously pink or peach, but other shades will appear to be more neutral. It is difficult to evaluate a color that's standing by itself, so look at several shades together for comparison. Put blobs of three or four colors on the back of your hand. Which ones have a pink or purplish cast? These are the cool shades, best for Winters and Summers. The warm shades, for Autumns and Springs, are the ones that look slightly yellow or peachy.

Once you've identified the cool and warm shades, you can narrow them down to the color that's right for you:

Winters: a cool, neutral shade, if you are olive, Asian or black; a slightly rosy beige if you have visible pink in your skin; a pale, sand color if you are very fair.

Summers: a pinkish beige if you have visible pink in your skin; a neutral cool shade if your skin is more beige than pink.

Autumns: a warm peach if you have ruddiness or lots of freckles; ivory if you are fair and slightly creamy; a warm "natural" beige if your skin is beige; golden beige if your skin is quite golden.

Springs: a warm peach or pinky peach, if your face is ruddy or you have "high coloring"; porcelain or ivory if your complexion is creamy and light; golden beige if your skin is darker and golden.

Choose the warm or cool foundation that most closely matches your natural skin tone. As a final step, you *must* test a foundation on your face, preferably on the jawbone. The skin on your wrist and hand varies tremendously from the skin on your face. Don't try to match the color to your cheeks, either, as they may be rosier than the rest of your complexion. Avoid "adding color" to your face with a foundation that is darker than your skin. You will have an unnatural line around your jawbone, and you will look older. Actually, a shade of foundation that is a smidge *lighter* than your skin makes you look more youthful. Give it a try, but don't go too light or your face will appear chalky.

When shopping, use the Foundation Test chart on the next page to help you choose the perfect color of foundation.

Once you have found your perfect foundation shade, you'll want to reevaluate it from time to time. The sun, your diet, the medications you take, tension, and your general state of health may affect your skin color and, in turn, the way your makeup looks. When tan, apply the same warm and cool principles, but select a darker shade of foundation.

FOUNDATION TEST CHART

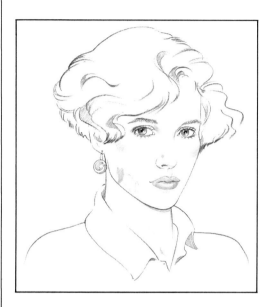

1. Using your season as a guide, select two or three shades of foundation that are in the right color range for you.

2. Making sure your face is clean and free of makeup, apply thin stripes of each foundation along your jawline with downward strokes.

3. Wait a few minutes and observe each shade as it dries. If possible, check the results in natural light. The wrong shade will "sit" on your face, leaving an obvious stripe. If the color is right, it will blend into your skin with the *edges* almost disappearing. If none of these shades is perfect, repeat the process. You may have to go on to the next makeup counter to try another brand.

4. Once you find the best color, remove the stripes and reapply it on your jawline, this time blending it in. It should be imperceptible.

5. When you think you have found the right foundation, apply it to your entire face right from the testers and wear it for a while. If it still looks great after an hour, you've made the right choice. If it has turned chalky, the foundation is either too light or too cool a shade for you. If it has turned orange, the foundation is either too dark or too warm a shade for you, or it contains too much oil.

CHOOSING THE RIGHT FORMULAS

Foundations come in three basic formulas: water-based, oil-based, and oil-free. Most of today's modern formulas are water-based liquids, creams, mousses, or cakes with a small amount of oil, designed to give you sheer to medium coverage. These foundations are suitable for most skin types and are designed to be worn over your moisturizer and other skin-care products. They are not meant to be substituted for proper skin care. A proper skin-care regimen will provide your skin with the moisture it needs so your foundation can be light and comfortable. Water-based formulas apply smoothly with a cosmetic sponge and are easy to work with.

If you have extremely dry skin, you may want to consider an oil-based foundation in which oil is one of the major ingredients. These foundations tend to have thicker coverage, which can accentuate wrinkles, but they do give extra protection to dry skin, especially in the wintertime or in cold climates.

Oily skins, especially those that break out, usually need an oil-free formula. Women with slightly oily skin may want to switch to an oil-free foundation in the summertime or in any hot, humid climate. Oil-free formulas do not spread easily, but they are a blessing for those women plagued with excessive oil. Apply them with your fingertips, let dry, and then "buff" your face with a dry cosmetic sponge. Because these formulas consist of mostly water and powder, the buffing technique works well to smooth out the application. Some brands are so thin they can be applied with a cotton ball before being buffed. An oil-free foundation cannot be used around the eye area as it is too drying. You will need to buy a second foundation with some oil content to apply around your eyes, or use a coverstick there instead. In either case, choose a similar or slightly lighter color.

To check the oil content of a formula, read the label. Ingredients are listed in order of predominance. In an oil-based formula, oil is the second or third ingredient (water is always first); in a water-based formula, oil is in the middle or near the end; an oil-free formula obviously has no oil.

You might also ask the salesperson what kind of coverage a product offers. If you have clear, beautiful skin, you need only a light, sheer coverage. To cover average skin with a few imperfections, medium coverage is desirable. Heavy formulas are best reserved for the stage, unless you have a major problem with skin discoloration. If you have problem skin, you may be tempted to reach for more coverage, but a heavy formula will both accentuate and aggravate raised blemishes and is best avoided.

Caution: Never add water to your foundation to make it more sheer. Water will not only change the chemical balance of your product, but may also add irritating bacteria. If you want sheerer coverage, apply your foundation with a dampened cosmetic sponge, or choose a lighter formula.

INGREDIENTS AND SENSITIVITIES

Foundations consist primarily of water, talc, oil, pigments, various additions to benefit the skin, preservatives, and, sometimes, fragrance.

Ingredients that benefit all skin types are aloe (a skin softener), soluble collagen (to maintain suppleness of the skin's outer layer), hyaluronic acid (to add moisture), hydrolized elastin (to enhance elasticity), and PABA (sunscreen).

If you have allergies or sensitive skin, choose foundations with almond, sesame, or avocado oils. These natural oils are known for their soothing properties and low level of irritation. Even though mineral oil is a natural substance, you should avoid it unless your skin is very dry, for its heaviness can make it hard for skin to breathe. Lanolin is an excellent emollient, but in large amounts it can irritate sensitive skin. Most foundations contain very little, however, so don't be scared off if it appears at the bottom of the list of ingredients.

If you are prone to acne, stay away from foundation containing oil (except perhaps as one of the last ingredients), fragrance, and detergents such as sodium laurel sulfate and laureth-4. In addition, some dermatologists feel that isopropyl myristate may exacerbate breakouts in acne-prone skin. This ingredient helps improve absorption of emollients, a plus for dry skin, but a potential problem for those who break out from excessive oil.

SPECIAL CONCEALING PRODUCTS

In addition to foundation, you may want to consider buying one of the special concealing products created to give additional coverage to problem areas: coverstick, color adjuster, or eye shadow base.

A *coverstick* is a spot concealer designed to minimize dark circles under the eyes, "smile lines" (shadows that run from the nose to the corner of the lips), the shadow between lip and chin, or the occasional blemishes nearly all of us suffer. A coverstick comes in a lipstick-type tube, or occasionally in a wand, in light, medium, and dark. I recommend buying a color as similar to your foundation shade as possible, or slightly lighter. A shade that is too light, applied under the eyes, will make you look like an owl.

When applying coverstick under the eyes, dot the coverstick on your under-eye brush and apply coverage just on the dark ridges where you need it. Applying concealer on the whole under-eye area will make your eyes look puffy. Blend by patting with your fingertip.

You can apply concealer *under* foundation, *on top* of foundation, or *by itself.* I prefer to apply it on top, and then pat to blend, for the most natural look. For a severe under-eye problem you may want to apply your concealer more heavily and then cover with foundation, but do pat the foundation on gently or you risk removing the coverstick. If you choose to wear coverstick alone under your eyes, be sure the color is compatible with your foundation.

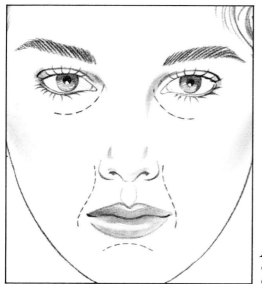

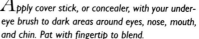
*A*pply cover stick, or concealer, with your under-eye brush to dark areas around eyes, nose, mouth, and chin. Pat with fingertip to blend.

Color adjusters are products designed for people with extremely ruddy (red) or sallow (yellow) skin. They are similar in texture to foundation, only thinner. The come in tubes, wands, or bottles, and are applied under foundation. Buy an aqua shade to neutralize ruddy skin; use a lavender shade to perk up sallow skin. For ruddiness, apply a thin coat with a cosmetic sponge just on the ruddy areas, usually the cheeks. For sallow skin, thinly coat your forehead, cheeks, and chin.

Eye shadow base is applied to the upper eye area, the lid, and the underbrow, and helps cover veins or very dark lids. In addition, it helps hold your eye shadow on all day, and prevents eye shadow from creasing. For this reason, many women like to use it on the upper eye area instead of foundation, even if they don't have a problem with veins or dark lids. It comes in a mascara-type wand, a tube, or a little pot, usually in one neutral shade. You apply it with the wand, your finger-tips, or a clean eye sponge applicator, and blend with your cosmetic sponge. You do *not* apply foundation on top of eye base. Black skins do not need this product for coverage, but may want a thin eye base just to hold the shadow on better. These thinner bases usually come in taupe, silver, or gold—almost transparent shades.

If you have a serious problem with scars or pigment discoloration, there are some specialized products available. Usually they are prescribed by dermatologists, but a few cosmetics companies carry such products. You'll have to ask. Lines that specialize in cosmetics for black skin often have pigment correctors, especially for lips.

APPLYING FOUNDATION

With all the elements assembled—your foundation, concealers, cosmetic sponges, and brushes—you're all set to start working makeup magic! Don't be daunted. It takes less than a minute to apply foundation. Add another minute if you want to use coverstick and eye base. Add a third if you need color adjuster. With practice, your whole routine, including powder, blush, eye shadow, mascara, and lipstick, will take no more than five to eight minutes. At night or for a special occasion you can spend more time fussing or experimenting with your makeup, but for work or everyday, it's a snap. So there's no excuse for ever leaving your house without your finished look!

Always apply foundation with a cosmetic sponge. Your fingers can stretch and pull your skin, and the application will be less even. A dry sponge gives a slightly heavier coverage. For a sheerer look, use a sponge that's slightly moist, but not wet.

Remember to just read and enjoy right now. All the instructions are summarized in the flip charts at the back of the book.

THE STEPS

1. (Optional) Apply *color adjuster* with a dry cosmetic sponge. Dot on the areas where needed, then pat and slightly blend with the sponge.

2. Dab *foundation* on the corner of your cosmetic sponge. Avoid dipping your fingers in the bottle, which can contaminate the contents.

3. Dot the *foundation* on your forehead, cheeks, nose, and chin, then smooth it evenly over your entire face with downward and outward strokes. (The hairs on your face grow downward.) Spread foundation only down to your jawline—the colors of your face and neck never match, so foundation on your neck will show. Blend the foundation carefully along your jawline so there are no rough edges.

4. With the corner of your sponge, gently work *foundation* into the area around your nose and under your eyes. If you don't plan to use eye shadow base, apply foundation to the upper eye area as well.

5. Lightly cover your mouth with the leftover *foundation* on the sponge. Too much foundation on the lips can cause your lipstick to run.

6. (Optional) Using your under-eye brush, dab *coverstick* under your eyes, only on the dark areas. Remember, don't apply coverstick to puffy spots or you'll call attention to them. Use the same method to minimize shadows around your nostrils or the smile lines around your mouth and in the hollow above your chin. Dot the coverstick lightly on your blemishes as well. Blend by patting lightly with your *clean* fingertip. The warmth of your finger will melt the coverstick so the edges will blend, but don't rub or blend it to the point that it disappears.

7. (Optional) Place a small dot of *eye shadow base* on each eyelid and blend it from your lids to your brows, using a sponge or your fingertip. Allow it to set for a moment before you open your eyes.

That's it! You're finished. See how easy it was? Now you have a choice. For a beautiful, basic everyday look, you can skip the following chapter and go on to the next easy step—powder. If, however, you want to spend some extra time learning the art of contouring your face, now's the time to curl up with Chapter 8, "Face Sculpting."

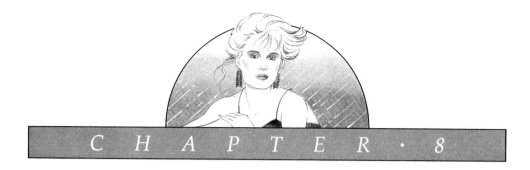

Face Sculpting

Face sculpting is the art of enhancing or minimizing sections of your face using the artist's principles of shadow and light to create illusions. Sculpting can slim your nose, minimize a heavy jaw or a double chin, widen your eyes, create high cheekbones, or even give you a temporary "facelift."

Sculpting is not for everyone. Some women don't need it and others don't want to fuss that much. And in the daytime, you must use a very light hand, as sculpting can look artificial in daylight. Still, you may want to try it if you're being photographed, appearing on TV, or going out for a glamorous evening.

Sculpting is always done after you apply your foundation and before you brush on powder. The two techniques involved are *highlighting*, or using light to accentuate, and *contouring*, or using shadow to create shape and to minimize.

To highlight you'll need a foundation or a coverstick one or two shades *lighter* than usual. For evening, you could even use a white or a pearly shade. To contour, you'll use foundation, coverstick, or tinted pressed powder in a shade slightly *darker* than usual.

For most sculpting illusions, a foundation or a coverstick will be your best choice for contour shades because they're the least obvious and the easiest to use. But for "lifting" your eyes, you'll need the tinted pressed powder, which you may also prefer for some of the slimming techniques as well. Choose a soft, neutral color slightly darker than your foundation. In buying a tinted powder, be guided by your season: *Cool* Winters and Summers should choose a slightly rosy beige; *warm-toned* Autumns and Springs, a more golden beige. You may have to go to a beauty supply house to find contour powder, as most cosmetic lines don't carry it.

Once you've assembled the proper tools and products, the keys to successful sculpting are a light touch and careful, even blending. In other words, don't overdo it!

Now determine the features you want to sculpt.

YOUR EYES

Eye sculpting is done on top of your foundation and regular concealers, including eye shadow base. To widen and "lift" your eyes, use your under-eye brush to place a medium-size dot of highlighter at the inner corner of each eye, on each side of the bridge of your nose. Gently press each dot for a few seconds to blend in the highlighter. Next, do the same thing at the outer corner of each eye. (*One exception*: If your eyes are very close together, omit the highlighter at the *outside*

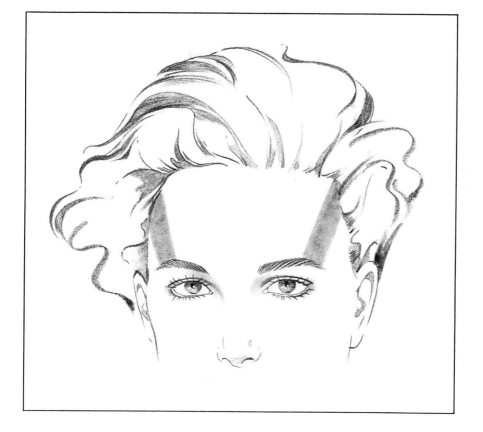

corners.) The highlighter will seem to "erase" the boundaries of your eyes, making them appear bigger.

To give "lift" to your eyes, apply *powder* contour shade just above the outside half of your eyebrow, sweeping it up to the hairline. You can use either your blush brush or your big, fluffy powder brush for a soft effect. You should not see much actual color, but rather a soft shading that will seem to lift the eye. Follow with your regular eye makeup (see Chapter 11).

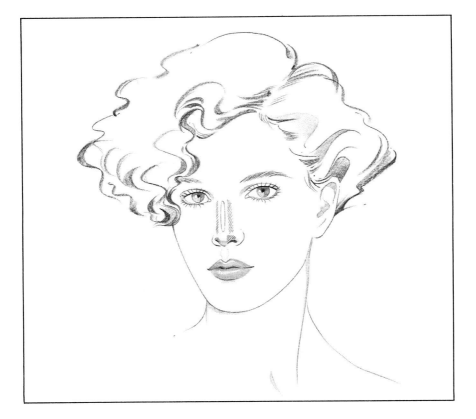

YOUR NOSE

To slim your nose, you will need both your highlighter and your contour shade, as well as a clean under-eye brush. With your highlighter, draw a line down the center of your nose and pat it with your fingertip to blend lightly. Next, draw a line with your contour shade down each side of your nose, again patting to blend. Make sure you don't leave any rough edges where the contour shade and highlighter meet. Now, to make the tip of your nose more angular, apply a touch of your contour shade in the bevels on either side of the tip of your nose. Finally,

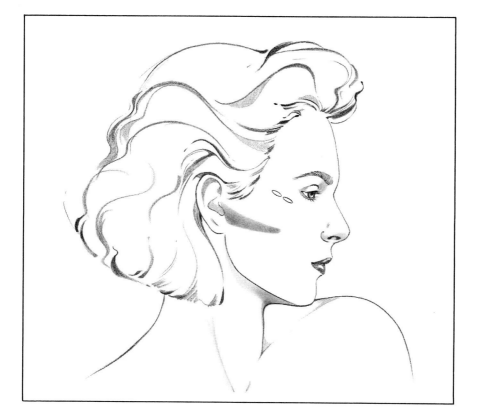

take a sponge still damp with your normal foundation and press it gently over your nose to soften the effect.

YOUR CHEEKS

You don't have to be born with the fashionably high cheekbones so many glamorous models have. Here's how they get them. First, find your cheekbones with your fingertips. With your under-eye brush, dot a line of highlighter along the top edge of each cheekbone up to the hairline, then gently pat with fingertips to blend. Next, take your contour shade and make a similar line of dots along the bottom edge of each cheekbone, in the hollow of your cheek, and blend once again. Now, lightly press your sponge, still damp with your regular foundation, over your cheekbones to soften the sculpting. If you want to intensify the effect, you can lightly dust your tinted contour powder just under your cheekbones, using your fan brush. Later, you will apply blush to the crest of your cheekbone.

If your cheeks seem sunken or your face too thin, you can "fill out" this area by applying your highlighter to the area *below* your cheekbone, and omitting it from above. Do not, however, apply the darker contour shade above the cheekbone, as it will make your eyes look sunken.

YOUR LIPS

Many of us have lips that are unbalanced, with one larger or smaller than the other. Here's how to correct the disparity.

First, cover your lips entirely with foundation to erase existing lip boundaries. Then, to bring out a small lip, take a clean under-eye brush and draw a thin line of highlighter along the outer edge of your lip, feathering lightly. To reduce a full lip, draw a similar line with your contour shade. You can also apply your lipstick or lip pencil a *teeny* bit outside your lip line on your thin lip and a bit inside the boundary on your full lip (see page 157). But be subtle. Your balancing shouldn't be noticeable.

After sculpting, follow with lipstick as usual (see Chapter 12).

YOUR JAWLINE AND CHIN

For a wide jaw (one that is broader than your cheekbones) or a bothersome double chin, you can use your contour shade either alone or combined with tinted powder. Simply blend the contour shade along your jawline and underneath your chin. For evening or photography, you may want to add another light brush of tinted powder. If you prefer, you can use the tinted powder alone for softer shading.

These are fun little tricks to play with on a rainy day or when you're in the mood to try for dramatic special effects. For everyday wear, you'll simply dust your foundation with a pouf of powder. Read on!

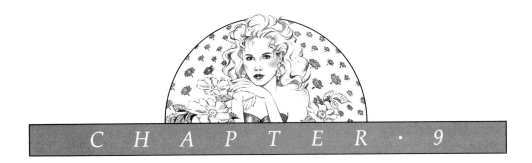

Powder

Once you've applied your foundation, concealer, and any sculpting products, you're ready for powder, the finishing touch. (If you use a moist blush, this too will go underneath your powder. We'll get to blush in the next chapter.)

We need powder for three reasons. First, it removes any tackiness from the foundation, leaving a smooth, dry finish on which to apply blush. Blush can "grab" or streak if applied directly to foundation, especially in hot or humid weather. Second, powder keeps your foundation fresh-looking all day. Third, and best of all, it gives your face a beautiful, matte finish that will bring you compliments on your wonderful complexion. Try powdering just one side of your face to see what a difference it makes!

Today's powder is extremely light and sheer, as far from the cakey kind our grandmothers wore as the ice chest is from the refrigerator. It will not accentuate wrinkles and can be applied to the eye area (eyes closed, of course).

Powder is for all skin types. If you're using an oil-free foundation, however, you won't need powder. Oil-free foundations consist of watered talc, so they will dry powdery. Once buffed, you will already have your smooth, matte finish.

CHOOSING THE RIGHT COLOR

Powder comes in shades similar to foundation colors. You can also buy a colorless, translucent powder suitable for any foundation; it simply disappears into the foundation, even on black skin tones. In addition, you will find powder in tints of pink, peach, lavender, and green, in both matte and iridescent finishes, as well as silver and gold in an iridescent finish only. Matte is for daytime, iridescent for night.

To choose a natural color, follow the same guidelines as for foundation: a rosy beige tone for the cool Winters and Summers, a golden tone for Autumns and Springs. Colorless, translucent powder, of course, is excellent for all seasons. I prefer it because it looks totally natural and you can't go wrong.

To wear tinted powders, again use your season's palette: pink or silver for the cools, peach or gold for the warms. Green and lavender powders are similar to color correctors. Lavender is for the sallow skins, green for the ruddies.

TYPES OF POWDER

There are two types of powder: loose and pressed.

Loose powder is desirable because it has no oils added to hold it together. It's the powder you will use at home to give you that wonderful, finished look. It applies easily with a fluffy brush or a soft puff, and you can apply as much as you like because any excess will simply brush off.

You can buy loose powder in a boxed container, but my personal preference is a shaker bottle, which allows you to sprinkle out just enough powder for one application into your hand. This method keeps loose powder from sifting all over your makeup table—both a mess and a waste. And because your powder brush touches only the dispensed powder, you never have to worry about adding bacteria to the container.

Pressed powder comes in a compact with a puff, is easy to carry with you, and is great for touch-ups. I always keep a compact of translucent pressed powder in my purse for spot touch-ups throughout the day. If you use a compact frequently, make sure you wash your powder puff often to prevent bacteria and oil from building up. Just slosh your puff through warm water and mild soap and then toss it into your dryer.

APPLYING POWDER

Powder is one step you won't mind adding to your daily routine because it's so quick and easy. You can't make a mistake, and the results are beautiful. Here, we'll apply regular, matte finish powder. You'll learn how to use iridescent powder in Chapter 13.

- To apply loose powder, begin by sprinkling a little powder into the palm of your hand. Dip your brush into the powder and shake off the excess. Then, using downward strokes to smooth your delicate facial hairs, brush the powder lightly on forehead, cheeks, nose, chin, and eyes, in that order. You want most of the powder on your face, less on the eye area. Give your face another light brushing, again with downward strokes, to remove any excess powder.

- To give your face an extra touch of radiance, you can dip your powder brush first in your blush, then in translucent powder, and stroke over your entire face. The hint of color adds a special glow.

- To make powder really stay on and keep your foundation "set" for hours, you can press the powder on with a firm powder puff or dry cosmetic sponge. Dip the puff into the powder and press it on your face, gently patting. Don't rub! Press and pat. If you feel you've overdone it and the powder looks thick, brush the excess off with your fluffy brush.

• To apply pressed powder, you can use a brush or the puff in the compact. Pressed powder tends to get hard, but you can loosen it by scratching a light X on its surface with your brush handle. Apply as with loose powder. To use the puff, simply pat it on where needed, repeating until any facial "shine" is gone.

Now your canvas is ready, so let's go on to the fun part—adding glorious color!

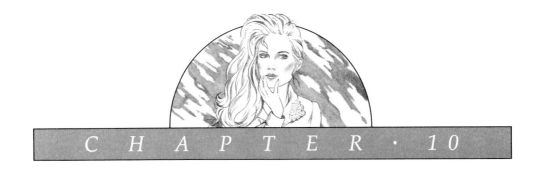

Blush

No other cosmetics item gives as immediate a result as blush. If you have little natural cheek color, blush will bring your face to life with a youthful, healthy glow. Even if your cheeks are rosy, blush will distribute the color more evenly, as nature tends to center the rosiness all in front. Blush comes in a wide range of forms, so you can easily find a type you like. Better yet, blush is available in a spectrum of colors appropriate for your season.

CHOOSING THE RIGHT COLOR

Knowing your season makes it easy to choose a blush that looks perfect on your skin tone and harmonizes with your wardrobe as well. Because you are choosing both blush and clothing colors from your season's palette, your makeup and wardrobe automatically go together!

You can wear one basic blush to blend with all your clothes, but you will look even better—and certainly have more fun—if you have several shades to coordinate more precisely with the range of colors in your wardrobe. A Winter can wear pink blush with her fuchsia blouse, but she will look more harmonious wearing fuchsia blush. Autumn's peach blush will blend with her terra cotta blouse, but why not go for the smashing look of terra cotta blush?

Using your season's Makeup Wardrobe Chart in Chapter 4 as a shopping guide, start with a basic, everyday blush and then add to your collection of shades as your budget allows. Remember, as you are shopping for a particular color—say, plum or peach, depending on your season—start with a medium color, and if it's too dark or light, go lighter or darker as needed. Blush colors are deceiving in the compact, and the color often looks quite different on your skin.

Here are some guidelines to help keep your shopping organized as you build your blush wardrobe:

Winters: For your basic color, look for a clear, medium pink or, if your skin is darkish, a burgundy. Black skins, especially, should consider burgundy their number-one basic. Be sure to choose shades that are true, rather than dulled. Your next blush purchases might be a soft, true red and a fuchsia, to go with those clothing colors. Last, add a plum to round out your wardrobe needs.

Summers: Start with a soft rose for your first blush. It's your most flattering shade and one that will match most of your wardrobe. Next, add a soft water-melon red and a soft fuchsia, to go with those special clothing colors. Don't go too bright on the red. You may want to try a cream or liquid rouge, which tends to go on softer than the powdered red blushes. Last, add soft plum to harmonize with your mauve, plum, and burgundy clothes.

Autumns: If your skin is medium to dark, you'll love a tawny peach blush for your everyday color; if you are very fair, try a lighter apricot shade. Next, add a salmon for the pinkish side of your wardrobe and a mocha shade to go with your browns and brown burgundy. Last, add a brick red to go with your reds and, depending on your coloring, either a chestnut or a brighter terra cotta for your rusts and pumpkins.

Springs: For your first purchase, aim for a clear salmon blush that's not too pink and not too orange. It's your perfect basic. Then add a peach or an apricot for the orange side of your wardrobe and a warm pink for your pinks. Last, you might get a soft shade of poppy red. Like Summer, you may want to choose a cream or liquid formula for sheer application. Be sure to avoid any brownish or tawny blushers. Spring needs clear colors to look her best.

CHOOSING THE RIGHT FORMULA

Blush comes in a range of forms—*powder, cream, gel, liquid,* and *mousse*—and under a variety of names, including *rouge, blush, blusher,* and *cheek tint. Rouge* is usually a cream, *blush* a powder, and *cheek tint* a gel or liquid. Each of these forms offers certain advantages. Some are especially suited to certain skin types; some are especially easy to apply; and certain types offer sheer coverage, ideal for bright colors. The form that's best for you will depend on a balance of all these factors. Let's look at each type.

Powder blush is the most popular and the easiest to apply. It comes in either a matte or frosted finish. Both matte and slightly frosted blush are suitable for day wear, but highly frosted blush is strictly for night.

With modern technology, pressed-powder blush has become so refined that it glides beautifully on *any* skin type. Look for a brand that feels smooth and silky when you rub it between your fingers. Grainy or chalky blushes will not go on as easily or look as sheer and natural.

Powdered blush is applied with a blush brush. Although most powder blushes come in a compact with a brush, you will find that the higher quality, natural hair brush in your at-home brush set (see Chapter 5) will give you the sheerest, smoothest effect. Use the brush in the compact for touch-ups. For most shades, you simply stroke your brush across the blush, tap off any excess, and apply. The pigments in red and deep-colored blushes tend to "grab," however, and you may need to dip your brush in loose powder first, then the blush, so the color will stroke on smoothly.

Cream rouge is applied with the fingers and is easy to use, but it must be well blended. Because of its fairly high oil content, cream rouge is not recommend for oily or acne-prone skins. Its creamy texture makes it a good choice for the woman with dry skin or one who wants a very subtle wash of color. You don't have to worry about a cream rouge being too bright, because you can blend it down to almost nothing. Choose a rouge that feels silky, not greasy to the touch.

In the past, cream rouge was often worn under powder blush to build up color intensity or to help the powder cling. With the quality of powder blush today, this is no longer necessary.

Creams come in either subtly frosted or nonfrosted shades. Frosts are best on younger skin (they may accentuate wrinkles) or in the evening to reflect candlelight.

To apply cream blush, place three or four dots of color along your cheekbone with your middle fingertip, then gently smooth and "feather" the blush with your ring and middle fingers until it is completely blended and no edges show.

Gels or *cheek tints* are sheer blushes that come in a tube or a pot and are applied with the fingertips. They are primarily water based, with little or no oil, so they are best on oily skin. However, because they contain so little oil, they also dry very quickly and can be difficult to apply. You have to dot them on one cheek at a time and blend deftly and quickly to avoid blotching. Mistakes with gels are harder to correct than with any other form of blush, and they will often stain your skin, making the color too bright. If the color is too heavy, go over it with a small amount of foundation on a dry makeup sponge (water will streak a gel), smoothing the entire area. When properly applied, gels have the benefit of looking very sheer and natural and will last for a long time. Gels are usually not frosted.

Liquid blushes, also called color rubs or washes, come in a bottle and are applied with the fingers. Like cream rouge, a liquid blush is easy to work with and provides sheer coverage. In fact, some of the washes are so sheer that you can use them all over your face for a subtle "sun-kissed" look. Liquid blushes are best on normal to oily skin.

Liquid blush comes both frosted and nonfrosted. The frosted shades are often sheer enough to wear even if you're older or have dry skin, and they can give you a fresh, dewy look.

To apply liquid blush, just dot it along your cheekbones and feather to blend with your fingertips, then smooth over with your cosmetic sponge, blending the edges well.

Mousses are sheer, light-textured foams that come in aerosol cans. They are suitable for all skin types, except the very dry. They, too, are applied with the fingers, which can be a tricky job. They tend to run and it's hard to place them properly, especially if too much foam pumps out. It's best to foam a small amount (about the size of a grape) into the palm of your hand. Then, using your fingertips, apply it thinly to dot and smooth it along your cheekbone. Blend the edges with a dry cosmetic sponge. If you want more intense color, apply a second coat rather than try to use a large dollop. Once you've learned to control them, mousses are natural-looking. They are not frosted and, once dry, can be blended at the edges with your contour brush.

To decide which blush formula is best for you, try on the testers at your local department store and see which are easiest for you to apply and which one feels best on your skin. If you're a true novice, buy a powdered blush. You can't go wrong. If you choose any of the moist blushes—cream, liquid, gel, or mousse—you will need to apply them directly on *top* of your foundation, *before* applying powder. Then follow with powder.

INGREDIENTS AND SENSITIVITIES

The primary ingredient in powder blush is talc, which is combined with coloring agents, preservatives, fragrance (sometimes), and oils and wax before it is pressed into form. Frosted blush includes mica or sometimes ground pearl to give it a shiny, smooth finish. Some powder blushes contain pure silk or cornsilk to smooth their application, but how smooth a blush feels is determined mainly by the degree of processing that the blush receives, rather than its ingredients.

Cream blush contains the same ingredients as powdered blush, but in different proportions—more oil and less talc. Liquids, gels, and mousses are water-based and tend to contain glycerin, or a similar substance, rather than oils, to make them spreadable.

Read the ingredients on the label to judge the oil or water content of the product. Remember, the ingredients are listed in order of predominance. Acne-prone skin will want to avoid mineral oil, unless it's one of the last ingredients in a powder blush. As with foundation, you will want to avoid isopropyl myristate, which may aggravate acne. Sensitive skins should avoid products containing fragrance or a high amount of lanolin. Sometimes a particular dye or preservative can cause a reaction. If your skin reacts to a product, you will have to be your own detective and try different brands and read labels until you catch the offending ingredient.

Be careful not to apply blush products near your eyes. Some may contain coal tar, which can cause blindness. I know many women who dab a touch of blush on the area above the eyes. Be sure to read labels if you plan on doubling your blush as an eye product. It can be dangerous!

APPLYING BLUSH

Once you've found a blush you like in your ideal basic color, you can quickly learn to apply it. The secret to a natural and flattering look is in the intensity and the placement.

As a rule of thumb, always apply just a little more blush than you think you need. The blush will look less bright once you've balanced it with eye makeup and lip color. And if you wish, you can always go back and adjust it. If your blush seems too bright, powder it or remove a little with your contour brush or a cosmetic sponge. If it's too pale, add a touch more. Balance is the key.

When wearing a brightly colored outfit, you may want to apply two shades of blush. First apply a soft color, and then dab a more vivid shade right on the crest of your cheekbone. You will get the intensity you need, but still look natural.

The right placement of your blush is just as important as the intensity. Applying blush too low can make your face look droopy. If you apply it too high, into the circles under your eye, you'll look as if someone punched you! Flattering placement is easy to achieve if you follow these simple guidelines.

THE STEPS

1. Looking directly into a mirror, apply blush along the cheekbone, starting right under the outer edge of your iris. You can find this spot by placing two fingers next to your nose—start there, outside your fingers. Blend the color out to the hairline at the tip of your ear. Most of the color should be on the crest of the bone, approximately at the outer corner of your eye.

2. Feather the color *slightly* downward into the hollow of your cheek, in a teardrop shape, but:

   • *Don't* go lower than the center of your ear at the outside, or below your nose on the inside.

   • *Don't* go closer to your nose than the outer edge of your iris.

   • *Don't* go into the circular area under your eye.

   • *Don't* go as high as your temple.

These are foolproof boundaries for proper placement!

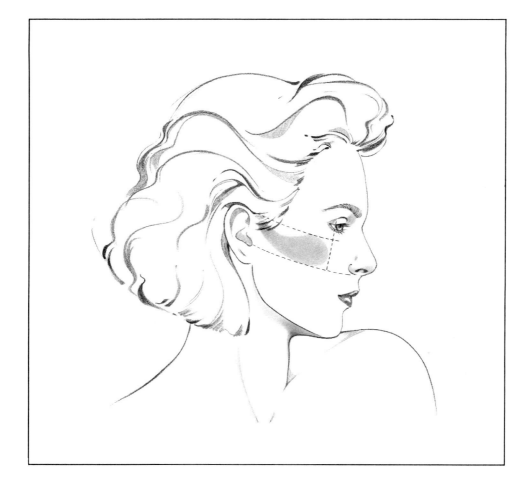

Note: If you used a contour shade in the hollow of your cheek, as in Chapter 8, then apply the blush just along the top of your cheekbone, blending downward into the contour shade.

3. Using your contour brush, which is slightly stiff, blend all edges so there is no distinct line where your blush ends.

SPECIAL TIPS

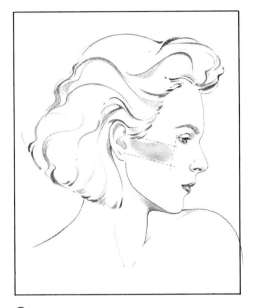

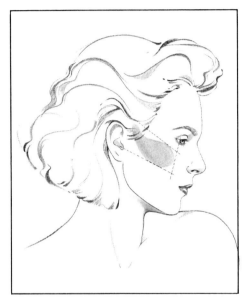

*I*f your face is quite narrow, you can widen its appearance by starting the blush at the outer corner of your eye and blending the color straight back to the hairline at the center of your ear.

*I*f your face is wide, slim its appearance by blending the blush slightly more upward toward the hairline just above each ear, and bringing it just a smidge lower than your nose, at the other end. You may also apply your blush in a wider band than those with narrow or average faces.

Using your Beauty Regimen chart at the back of the book as a guide, keep practicing until you get it just right. Before long you'll be able to apply your blush in seconds. You'll look great, and that's a happy way to start the day!

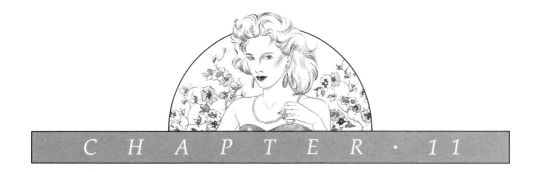

Eyes

Makeup has been enhancing beautiful eyes for eons; anthropologists think that the cavemen discovered copper and other metals in their quest for dramatic eye shadow. Cleopatra was famous for her glamorous eyes, as are the more recent beauties, Greta Garbo, Elizabeth Taylor, Sophia Loren, and Brooke Shields, all with magnificent eyes.

Although eye makeup is easy to apply, many women find it more intimidating than any other cosmetic. Most are comfortable with mascara and perhaps even a little eyeliner, but eye shadow is a puzzle. I didn't wear eye shadow for years, because I wasn't sure what color to buy, where to put it, or even why I should wear it. Now I'm a devotee. There is a vast difference between "natural" eyes with no makeup and "natural-looking" eyes with skillfully applied makeup. On the one hand, you are ignoring your eyes; on the other, you are enhancing their natural beauty! So let's make you famous for your beautiful eyes, too.

The purpose of eye makeup is threefold: to focus attention on your eyes by giving them definition; to accentuate the color of your eyes through flattering color choices; and to enhance the shape of your eyes through contouring. To accomplish these goals, eye makeup includes four different kinds of products: *eye shadow*, *eye liner*, *eyebrow definer*, and *mascara*. They come in various forms and colors, and work together to create a look you will love.

Here we will learn a basic, natural look—one you can use forever. As with clothing, eye makeup fashions come and go, but a polished, natural, attractive look will always be in style.

CHOOSING THE RIGHT COLORS

Knowing your season helps you select your perfect eye colors from the vast array of choices available at cosmetics counters. Eye products come in neutral shades as well as "color colors." Neutrals—the browns and grays—are the easiest to handle, and look natural. Generally, Winters and Summers should look for the cooler silver grays and blue-grays, or browns that have a grayish or cocoa tinge. Autumns and Springs will be flattered by warm browns, ones with hints of honey, gold, or copper, or yellow-grays.

For everyday wear, many women will prefer neutrals, always tasteful and almost foolproof to apply. But you can have fun with colors, too, and they can look nearly as natural as neutrals as long as they're applied with a light hand and are well blended. There is a vast, almost awesome array of colors available today—vibrant and discreet; intense and pale; mattes, frosts, iridescents, and even shadows with metallic glints. Matte or slightly frosted shades are your choices for daytime, with the sparkly ones reserved for night.

To sort through the wealth of makeup colors and find the ones best for you, begin by considering your season:

> *Winters* and *Summers*, look for *cool* shades, the ones similar to your wardrobe colors. Cool shades include taupe, pink, lavender, grape, purple, steel blue, navy, spruce green, mint, charcoal, and silver, in addition to your cool grays and browns.

Autumns and *Springs*, choose *warm* shades, like your clothing colors. Warm shades include ivory, peach, warm pink, sage green, olive green, yellow-green, warm violet, bronze, copper, and gold, plus your honey and coffee browns and yellow-greys.

Universal colors are champagne, aqua, teal blue, teal green, and periwinkle blue. These shades are on the border of both warm and cool and will blend with all the seasons' skin tones (but not necessarily with all eye colors, which we will discuss below). Another versatile color is turquoise, but I have included it only on the Winter and Autumn charts because it can be too dark for Spring and Summer.

Practice recognizing warm and cool eye shadow colors. If you line up six different shades of green eyeshadow, you'll see that some are warm, such as olive, sage and golden green; and others, such as spruce and mint (harder to find, by the way), are cool, devoid of a yellow cast. Go back to the makeup palettes on pages 21 to 27 and take a look at each season's green. See what a difference the undertone makes? Then look again at the eye color illustration on page 34.

Now that you know your range of shades, you need to consider the color of your eyes. The rule here is that makeup must either *match* or *contrast* with your eye color. Aqua blue eye makeup may be a fine choice, judging by your season alone, but if your eyes are grayish blue, it will clash. Instead of enhancing the beautiful color of your eyes, the mismatched blue will look garish. A steel blue closer to your eye color will be much more flattering. Similarly, yellow-green eyes need warm greens and olives, rather than blue green. Rose brown eyes need taupes and cocoa rather than bronze or coppery shades. Try a little dab of eye shadow on your lid, just above the iris. Don't blend it. Just see if the color clashes or blends with your eye color. If it doesn't match, try another shade. Now you see why there are so many different varieties of blues, greens, and browns!

Contrasting colors are much easier to select than matching colors. Grape, violet, and purple, for example, will harmonize with blue, green, and brown eyes alike. Brown eyes can wear the most shades well because brown is itself a neutral color.

The Eye Makeup Charts on pages 132 to 135 list your color options according to both your season *and* your eye color. You will want to experiment with shades to find your favorites.

With your colors in mind, let's look at the types of eye makeup you'll need. A basic wardrobe includes at least *one eyeliner* or *eye pencil, two or three shades of eye shadow*, and *one mascara*. You may also want to buy an *eyebrow definer* if your brows need filling in. We'll consider each item in turn, with the appropriate colors.

Eyeliners and Pencils
Eyeliners and pencils are used for definition. They make your eyes stand out and help your eyelashes appear wonderfully full and thick. You may be accustomed to black eyeliner, but many more shades are open to you and may, in fact, be more complementary. Neutrals look the most natural, but you can also try colors that match or complement your eyes, especially for evening. It often looks great to line your lower lid with a neutral, and your upper lid with a color similar to your eye shadow.

Select a color that is similar in intensity to the color of your eyes, lashes, and brows. If you are a blond Summer, say, with pale skin and blue eyes, the black or charcoal liner that brunette Winters can wear will be too harsh on you. You'll want to select a lighter shade—maybe a medium gray or slate blue—in the same cool range. By the same token, if you are an Autumn with dark coppery hair and deep brown eyes, pale sage green eyeliner will disappear on you. You'll need a deeper green or brown to offset your vivid coloring.

Eye Shadows
Eye shadows enhance both the color and the shape of your eyes, making them seem larger, more expressive, even dramatic. Once you know how to use shadows, you'll probably enjoy them more than any other makeup you wear. Because they come in such a wide array of colors, they offer the greatest potential for creativity.

Your first purchases will be a *highlighter* and one or two *contour shadows*. The highlighter is used to lighten and bring out areas; the contour shade is used to recess and reshape areas. If you have a lid that barely shows, for example, you will put highlighter on the lid. If the bony area above your eye is prominent, you will apply a contour shade there, to push the area back and give the illusion of a larger eye. We'll discuss how and where to apply these shadows later in this chapter.

For your basic, everyday look, purchase fairly neutral colors that flatter your eye color. These will go with everything in your wardrobe automatically. As you get more comfortable with eye shadow, you can add shades to your collection, to blend with the colors in your wardrobe. Just remember that you never want to add a color—regardless of your clothing—that doesn't flatter your eyes.

Again, the intensity of your eye shadow should be based on your coloring. You don't want to look garish with a color that's too bright or dark, or overly subtle in a color that disappears. A deep teal may be fine for a dark-haired Autumn, but a pale aqua shade will be better for a blond, fair Spring.

The Eye Makeup Charts will show you some attractive highlighter and contour color choices for your season. Combining the shadow colors is relatively easy, because your choices all come from your color palette of harmonious colors. You might, for example, combine a pink highlighter with grape and purple contour shades, or a pale gray highlighter with medium gray and steel blue shadows, if you are a cool season. Warm seasons can combine peach highlighter with copper and brown shadows, or ivory with medium brown and teal. Now is your chance to experiment and be creative. Some of your most surprising combinations may turn out to be your favorites. (One of mine is grape and teal.) Just remember to blend the colors well!

Mascara
Mascara colors and plumps up your lashes to make them look long and luxuriant. The basic shades are the neutrals—black, brown-black, and brown—but navy,

forest, spruce, and olive can look natural, too, because they dry dark. Black is best for Winters and darker Autumns; brown-black for darker-haired Springs and Summers; and brown for lighter Autumns, Springs, and Summers. You can try navy if you have blue or brown eyes; forest, spruce, or olive if your eyes are green or brown.

Brighter-colored mascaras are in vogue today, but they will undoubtedly be gone tomorrow. Though neutrals are a must for a well-groomed office look, the brighter colors, if used with care, can be fun for the young or the young at heart. Teal, aqua, violet, and other vivid shades can be applied to the entire lash or just to the lash tips. I like them best worn over a neutral, as a faint second coat, giving just a hint of color when the light hits your lashes. If you want to try colored mascaras, choose ones in shades that match your eye shadows.

Eyebrow Definers

Don't buy an eyebrow definer unless you really need it to feather in bare spots or to even the length of your brows. Not only are heavily drawn brows out of fashion, but your eyes will look larger if your brows are not too dark. Sophia Loren, for example, early in her career had dark, heavy brows (look at some of her early pictures), but over time she began to bleach them to a slightly lighter shade, and her intense, beautiful eyes really came to life.

If you decide you need an eyebrow definer, choose one that closely matches your brows and blends with the color of your hair. Test the color by drawing a line on your forehead—it's the best way to see if a color has any hidden tints, such as red, that might clash with your coloring. Summer or Winter blondes should look for taupes without any red tones, while Autumn and Spring blondes should choose light golden browns. If you're a Winter or Summer with darker hair and brows, try cool cocoa or charcoal browns; the warmer reddish or golden browns are for the redheaded or brunette Autumns and Springs. If your brows are gray, try taupe or a light gray pencil; if your brows are truly black, you can use a charcoal pencil.

THE EYE MAKEUP CHARTS

The following Eye Makeup Charts summarize your color choices. After you see which colors are best for you, according to both your season and your eye color, go back to your season's Makeup Wardrobe Chart in Chapter 4 and cross off any eye shadow suggestions that won't harmonize with your eye color. In other words, every color listed on your Makeup Wardrobe Chart won't necessarily suit you, even if it suits your clothes. For example, if you have Autumn green eyes and decide to wear a teal blue blouse, you cannot wear teal blue eye shadow because it will clash with your green eyes. Instead, wear a teal green or a green that blends with your eyes, or wear one of your brown or copper shadows. These will complement both your blouse and your eyes.

You will usually have to try on several versions of an eye shadow color to find the intensity that's right for you. For example, a grape shade in one brand may go on very dark, while another brand's grape may look soft and light when applied. You can't always tell by the way the color appears in the container. I've seen a teal that looks ultra bright in the pan go on the skin so softly you can barely see it. Try the colors on—it's the only way to tell if one is right for you.

Note, too, that some eye shadow colors blend into the skin so they look almost as neutral as brown or gray, while other shadows remain more "colorful." On the chart, I have marked the more neutral shades with an (N), to help you make your selection. In addition, some highlighters are very pale and blend into the skin, so they barely show. You don't really see color; they simply lighten the area. Other highlighters have a bit more color, and you can see a tint of green, pink, blue, or peach when they are applied. To differentiate between the two, I like to call the brighter highlighters "uplifters," because in small amounts they lift and brighten areas of the eye. Uplifters are usually too colorful to use on the entire eye area, but a dash applied just under the arch of the brow or in the center of the lid can add a wonderful touch of "light" to these special spots. I've marked the uplifters with a (U).

WINTER EYE MAKEUP CHART

Eye Color	Blue	Green Hazel	Brown
Highlighter	Champagne Pale Gray Taupe Pale Pink Pale Yellow Cool Pink (U) Cool Blue (U) or Aqua (U) Light Lavender (U) Mauve (U) Silver (U)	Champagne Pale Gray Taupe Pale Pink Pale Yellow Cool Pink (U) Mint (U) Mauve (U) Silver (U)	Champagne Pale Gray Taupe Pale Pink Pale Yellow Pink (U) Mint (U) Aqua (U) Mauve (U) Silver (U)
Contour Shades	Cocoa (N) Cool Gray (N) Grayed Purple (N) Navy (N) Steel Blue (N) or *Teal Blue (N) Purple Sapphire Periwinkle Blue	Cocoa (N) Cool Gray (N) Grayed Purple (N) Navy (N) *Teal Green (N) or Spruce Green (N) Purple	Cocoa (N) Cool Gray (N) Grayed Purple (N) Steel Blue (N) Navy (N) Spruce Green (N) Purple Sapphire *Teal Blue *Teal Green
Liners	Black (N) Charcoal Gray (N) Navy (N) Deep Purple Periwinkle Blue Steel Blue or *Teal Blue (best match with eye color)	Black (N) Charcoal Gray (N) Spruce Green (N) Deep Purple	Black (N) Charcoal Gray (N) Navy (N) Spruce Green (N) Deep Purple *Teal Blue

*Note that Teal Blue or Teal Green will look like a "color" on a brown eye, but more neutral on blue or green eyes.

SUMMER EYE MAKEUP CHART

Eye Color	Blue Hazel	Green Hazel	Brown
Highlighter	Champagne Pale Pink Pale Gray Pale Yellow Cool Blue (U) or Aqua (U) Cool Pink (U) Light Lavender (U) Mauve (U) Silver (U)	Champagne Pale Pink Pale Gray Pale Yellow Mint Green (U) Cool Pink (U) Light Lavender (U) Mauve (U) Silver (U)	Champagne Pale Pink Pale Gray Pale Yellow Aqua (U) Cool Pink (U) Mint (U) Mauve (U) Silver (U)
Contour Shades	Cocoa (N) Silvered Mauve (N) Cool Gray (N) Grape (N) Steel Blue (N) or *Teal Blue (N) Periwinkle Blue Lavender	Cocoa (N) Silvered Mauve (N) Cool Gray (N) Grape (N) *Teal Green (N) Spruce Green Lavender	Cocoa (N) Silvered Mauve (N) Cool Gray (N) Steel Blue (N) Grape (N) Spruce Green (N) *Teal Green *Teal Blue Periwinkle Blue
Liners	Navy (N) Medium Gray (N) Charcoal Gray (N) Steel Blue (N) or *Teal Blue (best match with eye color) Amethyst Periwinkle Blue	Medium Gray (N) Charcoal Gray (N) Taupe Brown (N) Spruce Green (N) Amethyst	Medium Gray (N) Charcoal Gray (N) Taupe Brown (N) Navy (N) Spruce Green (N) Amethyst *Teal Blue

*Teal Blue and Teal Green will look like neutrals on blue or green eyes, but will appear more colorful on a brown eye.

AUTUMN EYE MAKEUP CHART

Eye Color	Brown	Green Hazel	Blue
Highlighters	Champagne	Champagne	Champagne
	Ivory	Beige	Ivory
	Pale Peach	Pale Peach	Pale Peach
	Pale Golden	Pale Golden	Pale Golden
	Yellow	Yellow	Yellow
	Peach (U)	Peach (U)	Peach (U)
	Light Warm	Light Warm	Aqua (U)
	Green (U)	Green (U)	Light Violet (U)
	Aqua (U)	Gold (U)	Gold (U)
	Gold (U)		
Contour Shades	Coffee Brown (N)	Teal Green or	Coffee Brown (N)
	Olive Green (N)	Warm Green or	Golden Brown (N)
	Sage (N)	Olive Green (N)	*Teal Blue (N) or
	Mink (N)	Sage Green (N)	Putty (Warm
	Bronze (N)	Coffee Brown (N)	Gray) (N)
	Copper	Golden Brown (N)	Bronze (N)
	*Teal Blue (N)	Putty (Warm	Copper
	Teal Green	Gray) (N)	Periwinkle Blue
	Warm Green	Bronze (N)	
		Copper	
Liners	Brown (N)	Brown	Brown (N)
	Olive Green (N)	Forest Green (N)	*Marine Navy (N) or
	Forest Green (N)	or Olive Green (N)	*Teal Blue (best
	*Teal Blue	(best match with	match with eye
	*Marine Navy	eye color)	color)
		Teal Green	Violet
			Turquoise

*Teal Blue or Marine Navy will look neutral on a blue eye, more colorful on a brown eye.

SPRING EYE MAKEUP CHART

Eye Color	Blue	Green	Brown Topaz

Highlighters	Champagne
	Ivory
	Pale Peach
	Warm Pink
	Pale Golden
	  Yellow
	Peach (U)
	Aqua (U)
	Light Violet (U)
	Gold (U)
		Champagne
		Ivory
		Pale Peach
		Warm Pink
		Pale Golden
		  Yellow
		Peach (U)
		Light Warm
		  Green (U)
		Gold (U)
			Champagne
			Ivory
			Pale Peach
			Pale Golden
			  Yellow
			Peach (U)
			Light Warm
			  Green (U)
			Aqua (U)
			Gold (U)

Contour Shades	Honey (N) Golden Brown (N) Clear Warm Gray (N) *Teal Blue (N) Periwinkle Blue Bronze (N) Light Copper Violet	Honey (N) Golden Brown (N) Sage Green (N) or *Teal Green (N) or Warm Green Bronze (N) Light Copper	Honey (N) Golden Brown (N) Bronze (N) Sage Green (N) *Teal Green Light Copper Warm Green

Liners	*Teal Blue (N) or
	Turquoise or
	Slate Blue (N)
	  (best match with
	  eye color)
	Brown (N)
	Light Brown (N)
	Periwinkle
	Violet
		Brown (N)
		*Teal Green or
		Olive Green (N) or
		Sage Green (N)
		  (best match)
		Violet
			Brown (N)
			Olive Green (N)
			*Teal Blue
			*Teal Green
			Turquoise

*Teal Blue and Teal Green look more neutral on a blue or green eye, more colorful on a brown eye.

135

CHOOSING THE RIGHT FORMULA

Before you set out to purchase your eye makeup, you'll want to consider the various forms available.

EYELINER

Eyeliner comes in a *pencil, liquid,* or *powder* form. I prefer the pencil as it is made of wax and oil and can be "smudged" to look soft and natural. Be sure to choose one that is creamy so it won't pull the delicate tissue around your eyes. The drawback to pencils is that the color can run in hot weather, and they are too thick for women with very sparse eyelashes.

Liquids, applied with a brush, stay on well, but tend to create a harsh, continuous line that can be difficult to keep thin and straight. The key to success with liquid liner is choosing a color that is not too dark, and applying with a thin, good-quality eyeliner brush. Liquids work especially well for women with crepiness on the lids.

You can also use powdered eye shadow to line your eyes. Apply it with a thin, moistened eyeliner brush. It dries to a soft, powdery line that can be blended with a dry under-eye brush. (You can also draw the line with dry eye shadow powder and a dry eyeliner brush. It won't stay on as long, but will look extremely natural.) In warm or humid weather, eye shadow can be the best choice for eyeliner, as it doesn't contain much oil and won't melt from the heat. Moistened, it is also an excellent choice for women with crepiness on the lids or women with sparse lashes. The thin brush places the liner close to the lashes, and the "powdery" line looks natural.

EYE SHADOW

Eye shadows come in *pressed powder* form, as well as in *creams, liquids* and *crayons.* Some of the new crayons are called *powder crayons,* containing the same ingredients as pressed powders but molded into the shape of a fat crayon.

Shadows come in matte, frosted and iridescent formulas. Matte or lightly frosted types are best for daytime; frosts or iridescents for evening. Unless you're very young, you should avoid highly frosted shadows entirely, as they accentuate crepiness.

Powdered shadows are the most popular and easiest to control. Their talc base is mixed with oils so they glide smoothly on all skin types. As with blush, the shadow should feel silky, never chalky or grainy, when you rub it between your fingers. Powdered shadows are applied with a brush or an eye sponge. The brush is used for lighter application and for general blending, the sponge for heavier coverage and for blending stubborn edges.

Cream eye shadows are sometimes preferred by women with dry or aging skin, since they contain more wax and oil and will minimize crepiness. Creams are not recommended for oily skin, as the color tends to slip off and collect in the crease of the eye.

Usually applied with the fingertips, creams can be hard to place correctly and blend evenly. Even the types that come in a tube with a wand are difficult to control. If you like cream shadows, try dotting them on with your fingertip, the tip of the wand, or a clean under-eye brush and then blending them with a dry eye shadow brush to place them more precisely and smooth the edges.

Eye crayons, whether creamy or powdered, can be "drawn" on and then blended with a clean, dry eye-shadow brush or your stiffer contour brush. They are easy to control, and the powdered ones blend especially well. I don't recommend using the creamy eye crayons on a daily basis, because you must apply a fair amount of pressure to spread them with your brush, and the tugging can stretch your skin, encouraging wrinkles.

MASCARA
There are *liquid, cake,* and *cream* mascaras. Liquid is the most popular and comes in regular, water-resistant, and waterproof forms. Regular mascara is fine, but it will run if your eyes water. I like the water-resistant type the best. It won't streak off during aerobics class, yet can be removed easily, even with soap and water. Waterproof mascara is best reserved for the beach or special occasions, as it makes your lashes very stiff and can be removed only with a special makeup solvent. (However, if your bottom lashes tend to smudge easily, which they do on women with short lashes that grow close to the skin, waterproof mascara on the lowers is worth the extra trouble.)

Liquid mascara is easy to apply. It comes in a tube with a wand that often has a little brush on the end to help separate the lashes as you stroke it on. Some liquid mascaras, called *lash builders*, have added nylon or rayon fibers that cling to your lashes, making them look thicker. They're great if your eyes aren't sensitive or you don't wear contact lenses. Otherwise, the little fibers can be irritating.

Cake mascara comes in a little compact and is applied with a wet brush similar to a tiny toothbrush. Because these are water based, they run very easily. Creams come in a tube, similar to toothpaste, only smaller. They are applied with a tiny brush also, but the cream is messy and harder to control than liquids and cakes. Creams do, however, give your lashes a soft, silky look.

EYEBROW DEFINERS
Eyebrow color comes in pencil or pressed-powder form. The powders are especially nice because they feather on with a tiny, stiff brush for a soft, natural look. If

you prefer a pencil, be sure to keep the point short and sharp so you can apply it lightly.

INGREDIENTS AND SENSITIVITIES

Eye shadows contain almost the same ingredients as blushes, but with different colored pigments. In addition, shadows exclude any ingredients dangerous to the eyes, such as coal tar dyes. As with blush, the powdered products are primarily talc, with wax and oil; the creams and liquids have more oil, less talc.

Of all your makeup, eye products are the most likely to trigger allergies or irritations. If your makeup is bothering your eyes, first look to your mascara and then to the shadows and liners. Avoid using each product in turn for a day or two, and if you find that the problem subsides, try replacing the offender with one from a hypoallergenic line or a brand containing different ingredients.

The additives most likely to spark reactions are fragrances (which most eye products avoid), preservatives, and cosmetic detergents, as well as certain colorants and oils. If you've been having trouble, steer clear of brands containing quaternium-15, thimerosal, or phenyl mercuric acetate (preservatives); aluminum powder, guanine, or carmine (color additives); sodium laurel sulfate (a detergent); and lanolin. Sensitive eyes should also avoid "lash-building" mascaras that have added synthetic fibers.

Be aware that some irritations are caused by you. You must keep your eye makeup and applicators clean. Never use a mascara for longer than six months, as it is the product most likely to breed bacteria. If your eyes are sensitive, avoid putting color near your tear ducts, the part of the eye most susceptible to irritation. And don't line the rims of your eyes inside your lower lashes. It is easy to scratch and irritate your eye, and the waxes and oils can settle into the socket of your eyeball.

Note, too, that not all problems stem from eye makeup. One friend of mine wasted two weeks looking for the cause of her suddenly swollen and puffy eyes. She spent a small fortune on new brands of eye shadow, but it seemed that she was allergic to all of them. After much discomfort and expense, she finally found the culprit—her eye makeup remover.

Spring pollens, summer grass, and winter molds can make your eyes extrasensitive, red, and itchy. If you suffer from hay fever and other seasonal allergies, give your eyes a rest from eye makeup for a few days during the especially bad periods.

APPLYING EYE MAKEUP

Now you've assembled your eyeliner, highlighting and contour shadows, mascara, and eyebrow definer, if you need one, and you're ready to learn to apply them. Your eyes should be prepared, as we discussed in the chapter on foundation, with eye shadow base or foundation. Expect some exciting results!

EVALUATING YOUR EYES

Start by evaluating your eyes in the mirror. Can you see the lid, or is it completely hidden when your eyes are open? Visually divide your eyes into two parts—the *lid* and the *brow/orbital bone*. Your crease is the dividing line. These are the two areas where you will apply shadows or highlighters to contour your eyes. See if you have more brow, more lid, or approximately equal amounts of each. As when contouring your face, you'll be using light shades to accentuate some areas and medium to dark shades to downplay others. Wherever you have the most room, you'll apply the contour shade; wherever you have the least area, the lighter shade. In all cases, you'll want to add definition to the outer corners of your eyes.

Study your eyes carefully so that in the steps that follow you can determine the most flattering placements for your makeup. While there are endless variations on eye shapes, I have found that the following four types of eyes are most common:

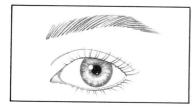

Proportioned: Lid and brow area approximately equal. On the proportioned eye, the lid and brow bone are balanced. Usually you have a bit more brow area than lid, but the lid shows. Here you will highlight under the arch of your brow, contour the shape of your orbital bone above the crease, and use a soft shade on your lid to enhance your eye color. If you have a lot of lid that shows *and* a lot of brow area, you'll follow the same principles, but you won't use bright colors.

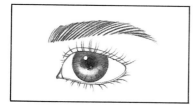

Little or no lid showing, more brow area. This type of eye has little or no lid showing, with a wider brow area. Asian eyes should consider themselves in this category, as should those with hooded eyes or prominent orbital bones. You will apply a pale highlighter to the lid to bring it out and a darker contour shade above the crease to help create balance.

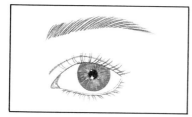

Little or no lid showing; small brow area. This eye has very little space on which to apply eye makeup. On this type of eye you will apply a light shade on both the lid and the brow area. Your goal is to visually expand the area between your eye and eyebrow.

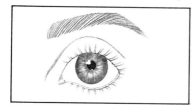

Prominent lid; small brow area. Here a lot of lid shows and is often a larger area than the brow bone. You will use a medium neutral shade on the lid to push it back and "expose" more of the iris, and a paler color on the brow and orbital bone to lift and open that area.

STEP 1: EYELINER

First, you'll apply your *eyeliner*, to define your eyes and to make them appear larger. You apply liner before eye shadow for two reasons. First, a creamy eye pencil won't go on smoothly over powdered eye shadow. Second, the application of eye shadow will help to soften and blend the liner, for a more natural look.

With a freshly sharpened pencil (or with liquid liner or moistened powder eye shadow) draw a thin line, as close to the base of the lashes as possible. Try to color in between the lashes so they'll look thick and luscious. Be careful not to pull or stretch the delicate skin around your eye. If your eye pencil is too hard or dry, swish it across the heat of your blow drier for a second or two, and it will become creamy.

For the proportioned eye, line the outer half of your upper and lower lids, feathering a smaller amount of liner towards the nose, to prevent the line ending abruptly. Emphasizing the outer half will "widen" your eyes. Some proportioned eyes have a lot of lid showing, as well as lots of brow. Use a neutral, rather than a bright color on this type of lid.

If little or no lid shows and you have either a large or small brow area, line the entire lower lid, to emphasize the bottom of your eye, but line only the outer third of your upper lid, to keep it "open" and make your eye look bigger. Lining the upper lid will close in your eye.

If your lid is prominent and you have a small brow area, line the entire upper lid almost to the tear duct, to recess the lid a bit, but line only the outer third of your lower lid, feathering the edge so it doesn't end abruptly. Use a medium neutral, rather than a dark or bright color. Then blend the line to soften it. Be subtle. Everything shows on your type of lid.

Now blend. Work the edges of your liner with an eye sponge or a clean under-eye brush until they grow soft and fuzzy. If the brush seems to spread out the liner too

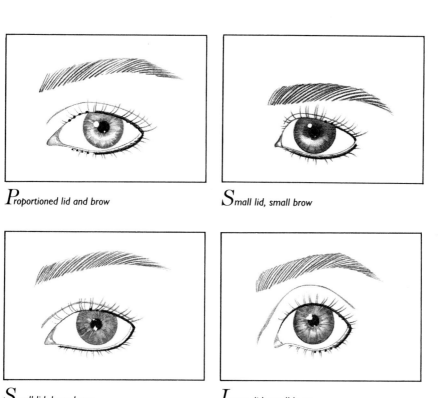

*P*roportioned lid and brow

*S*mall lid, small brow

*S*mall lid, large brow

*L*arge lid, small brow

much, try the sponge, which will remove any excess. (A cotton swab works, too.) What you're aiming for is a natural look—a barely perceptible rim of liner.

Set your liner by applying the same color of powdered eye shadow on top of it to keep it from smudging. (If you used black liner, set it with one of your dark eye shadows.) Do this with a clean under-eye brush, turned sideways to get a thinner line. You can skip this step if you used moistened eye shadow powder as your eye liner.

Special tip for sparse lashes: If you have few or no eyelashes, you cannot use an eye pencil. No matter how sharp, the pencil will create a line that will be too thick and obvious. Instead, dampen your tiny eyeliner brush and run it across a neutral shade of pressed eye shadow. Choose a color that is not too dark. Dot the color along the base of your eyelashes, rather than drawing a solid line. You just want to give your eyes a little definition. When dry, blend slightly with a clean under-eye brush turned sideways.

STEP 2: EYE SHADOW

Here is your chance to shape and lift your eyes, creating balance and proportion.

THE STEPS

Using your eye sponge, cover your entire eye area, from upper lashes to brows, with a matte or very slightly frosted highlighter. *If your lid is prominent*, don't apply highlighter on the lid; apply it only on the brow area down to the crease. You don't want to bring out the lid any more. For now, just leave it natural, with the foundation or eye shadow base. (See illustration A.)

With your angle brush, apply a dark to medium contour color on the outer third of

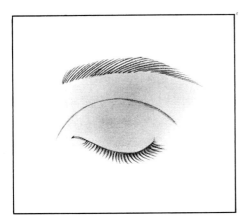

$A.$ First cover your entire eye area with highlighter. If your lid is prominent, cover only the brow area, not the lid.

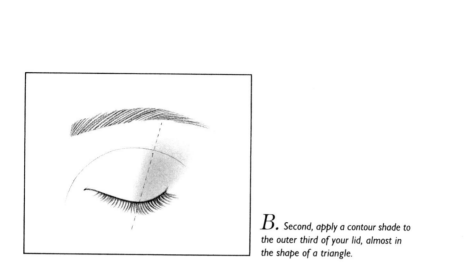

B. Second, apply a contour shade to the outer third of your lid, almost in the shape of a triangle.

your lid, almost in the shape of a triangle. Tap excess powder off your brush before applying, so the color won't "grab" and be too dark. This color can be neutral or more colorful, as it won't show much when your eye is open. Here's where you can have fun with colors. *If your lid is prominent*, don't use a bright color. (See illustration B.)

Next, you'll contour the orbital bone above the crease, using a medium color or neutral. You can use the same color you used on your outer lid if it's not too dark, but most women should not wear a light or highly frosted color on this area because paleness will bring it forward. You need shading to push back the orbital bone, letting your eye shine out. *If you have a small brow area*, you are the exception to the rule and will use a lighter shade on your brow area.

With your angle brush, again tapping off excess powder before applying, sweep the color from the *outer* edge of your eye inward, going all the way across the bone. Start the contour color just above the crease, blending slightly into the crease to look natural. Be sure you apply the shadow high enough onto the bony area. If it is too low and near the crease, your eyes will look sunken. Be careful, too, not to apply the shadow too low at the outer edge of your eye, or your eye will look droopy. Think of an imaginary line from the outer corner of your eye to the end of your eyebrow, and use this as your boundary.

For the proportioned eye, apply your contour shadow just above the crease, from the outer eye to the inner, concentrating most of the color on the outer two thirds of the orbital bone. As an extra touch, you can then apply an uplifting shade to the inner two thirds of your lid and just under the arch of your brow. If your lid shows a lot, skip this last step.

If little or no lid shows and you have more brow area, bring the contour shadow up higher in the center and extend it a bit closer to the nose, creating almost a semicircular shape. Having shadow higher in the center will "open" the eye and prevent a droopy look at the outside edge. You can, if you like, place a dot of uplifter over the center of your pupil, close to your lashes. Use a color similar to your eye color, or pink or silver for brown-eyed Winters and Summers, peach or gold for brown-eyed Autumns and Springs. Don't blend the dot much. The purpose is to make your eye look bigger by extending the "iris" upward a bit.

If little or no lid shows and you have a very small brow area, apply a pale color to the entire brow area, from crease to brow, instead of a contour shade. You don't need to push your brow bone back. Choose a color similar to your eye color, or use a pink or pale gray for cool seasons, peach or golden yellow for warms. You can then sweep a little of the color on your outer lid upward at the corner, toward the end of your eyebrow. Then, if you like, you can place a dot of uplifter on the center of your lid right over your pupil, close to the lashes. Don't blend it much. This dot will catch the light as your eyes move, and make the iris look bigger.

If your lid is prominent and you have a small brow area, you will apply a pale shade across the entire orbital bone, blending it toward the eyebrow. Now brush a little of the darker eye shadow from the outer corner of your lid up toward the end of your eyebrow, feathering it at the outer edge of your orbital bone. Finally, apply a subtle, medium neutral to the inner two thirds of your lid, to recess your lid. (If your crease is dark and sunken, stop the shadow short of the crease. This trick will help make your lid appear smaller, your brow larger.)

Now blend the shadow with your fluff brush until the edges are soft and the shape

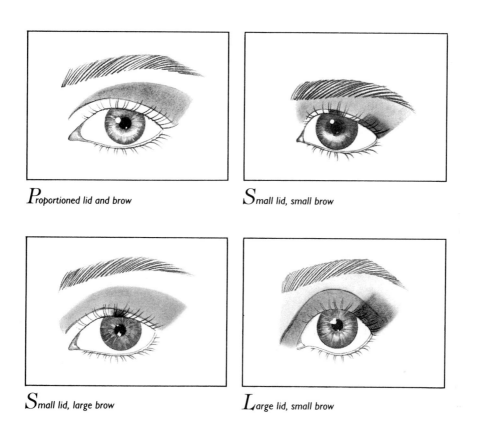

*P*roportioned lid and brow

*S*mall lid, small brow

*S*mall lid, large brow

*L*arge lid, small brow

on your orbital bone is flattering. For stubborn edges, use your contour brush to blend. Keep your eyes open while looking in the mirror and blending. This way you can adjust the shape and check your boundaries. If, at this point, you feel your eyes need brightening, apply a touch of eye shadow that is similar to the color of your blush right on the crest of each orbital bone. Use your fluff brush for subtle application. (You can use blush as long as you are *sure* the ingredients are safe for the eye area.)

Next, take your contour brush and lightly blend the entire area, using upward and outward strokes, from lid to brow. Blend until the intensity is just right and the edges are smooth. (If you wear glasses, allow the color to be more intense.)

Dust the entire area lightly with translucent powder to set your shadow and help it last all day.

STEP 3: MASCARA

For luxurious lashes, apply two coats of mascara to *all* your lashes, top and bottom. A few people will have to skip the bottom, for their lashes grow so close to the skin that their mascara always smears.

To coat your top lashes, look into the mirror, tip your head back slightly, and stroke on the mascara with your wand. Twirl the wand up and out to cover the lashes completely from the base to the tips.

To apply mascara to the bottom, tilt your head forward and twirl your wand down and out until the lashes are evenly covered. You may find it easier to use your wand vertically, applying the mascara with the tip of the wand with little downward strokes.

Comb your lashes with your brow/lash brush to separate them and to remove any clumps of mascara. Allow to dry for a few seconds.

Dust your lashes lightly with powder to thicken them before you apply your second coat.

Apply a second coat to top and bottom. (But don't dust with powder this time!)

To correct mistakes, dot the misplaced mascara with a cotton swab dipped in non-oily eye makeup remover.

STEP 4: EYEBROWS

Eyebrows frame your eyes, so you want them to look balanced. If you have kept them well shaped through judicious plucking, you may not have to do anything other than brush them into place with your brow/lash brush. But some of you will need to fill in bare spots or compensate for short or unequal brows, or thinner brows that are extremely sparse. Use the same guidelines for length that you used when you plucked your brows (see page 90). Please use caution. Remember, overly penciled brows can ruin your looks.

Take your pencil or brush dipped in pressed powder and feather the color on with quick, short strokes, to simulate little hairs. Never draw it on—a harsh line will be too obvious and will spoil the natural look you're trying to achieve.

Finish by brushing your eyebrows up and out with your brow/lash brush. If your brows need a bit of coaxing, use a touch of mustache wax on the brush first.

Voilà! See what a difference eye makeup makes? It takes practice, but it's well worth the trouble. Once you learn the routine, you'll be able to apply your eye makeup in three or four minutes, and with the right colors, you'll have "naturally" stunning eyes every single day!

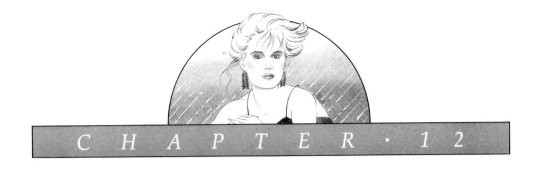

Lips

Although we communicate with our eyes, our lips do most of the talking. A woman's smile is the first thing people notice about her face. And surely the most sensual part of a woman's face is her lips. At least they can be, with properly applied lip color!

Some women are blessed with natural lip color. Lucky you, if you're one of them. Some of us, however, have almost no rosiness in our lips, and really need that touch of color to give us a healthy, vibrant glow.

There are three main types of lip products: *lipstick*, *lip gloss*, and *lip pencil*. Lipstick is my favorite because it gives excellent coverage and you have more flexibility and fun with colors. Gloss is sheer, can be tinted or colorless, and adds shine. It can be used to top off lipstick or can be worn alone, if you just want a faint hint of color. Lip pencils are essential accessories, used to outline your lips and to keep lipstick in place and fresh looking all day.

CHOOSING THE RIGHT COLOR

Like blush, lipstick should complement both your skin tone and your clothing.

Again, you can start with one or two basic colors to blend with your wardrobe, and gradually add a collection of shades in your season's palette that will more exactly match the variety of colors in your clothing.

Knowing your season makes it easy to know what colors you want; finding the colors in the store is harder. You may have to try several brands to find the perfect shades, but shopping and experimenting can be fun, and the right colors will make a world of difference in your appearance.

I strongly suggest that you take a friend shopping with you if you are at all unsure how to judge what's best on you. Remember to periodically update your look. Some women go for years wearing a lipstick that is too light, because that's what they wore in high school. Bear in mind, too, that as we age, nature fades our skin tones, hair, and eyes, and a color that was wonderful in our thirties may become too bright later on.

To shop for lipsticks, start by looking through the tester unit for cool or warm colors, depending on your season. Winters and Summers should scout for *cool pinks and reds*, rather than orange and peach shades. Autumns and Springs should stick to *warm* peach, coral, or peachy pink shades, avoiding hints of blue. To help you choose, compare cool blue-pinks, blue-reds and rose shades with warm yellow-pinks, orange-reds, and peaches. Today, luckily, some companies arrange their testers in warm and cool sections, to make your shopping easier.

After you have identified your range of colors, you need to select the color value that is best for you. Here's where the Color Me Beautiful Shopping System really works! You'll be amazed at how quickly you can select the perfect color. First, decide which color you are choosing—pink *or* plum *or* peach *or* red. In other words, don't try to select all your lipstick colors at the same time. Then, line up the lipsticks you're considering, from light to dark, and try on the shade that seems *medium* bright. If it is perfect, you're in luck. If it's too bright, try on the next lighter shade; if too light, try on the next deeper or brighter shade. Repeat this with each color you are selecting. You may not find all your colors at the same counter. Remember, if a particular brand doesn't have the right intensity for you, move right on to the next counter.

Balance the color of your lipstick with the depth of your coloring. A color that is perfect for a blond, fair Autumn will be too pale on a vivid, brunette Autumn. A vivid fuchsia lipstick that flatters a Winter will be overwhelmingly bright on a light-haired Summer, who instead needs a soft fuchsia.

Your lips themselves affect the desired intensity of your lip color. If your lips are either extra-full or thin, stick with fairly soft colors. Bright shades will accentuate either extreme. If you have vivid natural lip color, choose a shade that looks fairly soft in the tube. Your lips will intensify the color and it will look brighter once it's on. Or, choose a sheer formula that is slightly transparent. You may even want to just line your lips with a pencil that matches their natural color and fill in your lips with gloss.

Here are some guidelines for each season. Again, take your blank Makeup Wardrobe Chart with you so you can fill in the brand and color of your favorites. If you can't spend the money to buy all the colors you want, you will have the names written down for a future shopping trip.

LIPSTICK

Winters: Winters aim for clear, bright shades. Some Winters need softer colors if their lips are quite rosy. If you have lots of lip color, try a sheer berry color; for pale lips, try a medium pink or a raspberry. Next, test a slightly frosted pink to see if the vibrancy is better on you. Whichever you choose, your pink, raspberry, or berry lipstick will be your mainstay for everyday, and will complement the majority of the colors in your wardrobe.

After you've found the pink you love, look for a luscious red. If your hair is very dark, you can probably wear a true red or blue-red. (Avoid orange-reds; they're not for you!) Lighter Winters might try a softer, geranium color. If you are afraid of red, find a sheer tint or gloss; it will still be red, but you won't feel like Vampira. You do need *some* red to go with your red clothes.

Next, you will enjoy a fuchsia. There are so many varieties of fuchsia, you'll probably need to try a soft one, a bright one, and a dark one, to see which is the best depth for your coloring. If you don't own any clothing in fuchsia, you could skip this color, but fuchsia also looks beautiful with your emerald green, royal blue, and purple.

Eventually you'll need a burgundy or plum to go with your burgundy clothing. Most black Winters look gorgeous in burgundy lipstick and can wear it as an everyday color. If burgundy is too strong for your skin, find a sheer or a lightly frosted shade. Or, try using burgundy pencil to cover lips completely, and then glaze them with a pale plum or raspberry lipstick. You'll get the color you need, but softer.

Summers: Start with a soft-to-medium rose or pink. If your lips need color, go for brighter shades, but if your lips are pink to start with, you may prefer a dusty rose. A delectable pink will be your basic lipstick color and will go with almost everything in your wardrobe. You will probably want several pinks, ranging from rose pink to some blue-pinks, for variety.

Now you'll want a red to wear with your red clothing. Choose a watermelon shade or a soft blue-red (or both). These may be hard to find. If you can't get the soft red you need, instead choose a cool shade of red that's too bright and tone it down by applying pale pink or a "white" toner over it. Or, choose a tinted red lip gloss. Avoid all orange reds; they'll clash with your cool skin tone.

Fuchsia is an especially nice choice for your next shade. Many Summers find that fuchsia is one of their best colors because they have so much pink in their skin. Look for a soft or even slightly frosted shade.

Last, choose a soft plum, wine, or mauve shade. Keep the color fairly light, not heavy. This lipstick will be beautiful with the burgundy, plum, and mauve side of your wardrobe.

Autumns: Choose your colors with special care, as Autumns vary more than any other season. If your hair is light, you will look best in soft, muted shades of tawny peach or cinnamon. You may even find that a brownish honey color is your best shade for everyday. Brown-haired and red-haired Autumns will prefer terra cotta tones in more intense shades for their basic, everyday lipstick.

Next, you'll need a lipstick that verges toward pink to wear with the salmon and salmon pinks in your wardrobe. Look for a tawny salmon, which will give you a touch of pink without straying into the cool range. Avoid all blue-pinks and fuchsias; they are much too blue for your warm skin tone.

Now choose a red to go with the red side of your wardrobe. If you look best in muted colors, look for a brick red, one with a slightly brownish tone. If you need brightness, select an orange-red. If you are light-haired and fair, try a sheer formula or a lip gloss.

Next, you'll want an orange or an orange-coral to wear with your brighter outfits. Vividly colored clothing needs a bright lipstick for balance. Many Autumns will do well with a burnt orange or pumpkin lipstick, but some—redheads, especially—look terrific in true orange (see Sharon, page 24). You might also try creating some beautiful coral shades by combining red with a lighter peach or the "yellow" lipstick toner most brands carry.

Finally, you may want a mahogany or mocha lipstick to wear with your rich browns or brownish burgundy clothing. Choose a deep shade or a soft muted color, depending on which intensity is most harmonious on you. Black Autumns look especially terrific in a rich mahogany shade, and may prefer it as their basic, everyday lipstick.

Springs: The most versatile lip color for a Spring is a clear salmon. Because it is between pink and peach, it blends well with all your wardrobe colors and is a great basic. Some blond Springs, however, love a pink lipstick and will prefer it as their everyday color. Other Springs, the redheads, often prefer peach as their basic. Whichever you choose to start with—salmon, warm pink, or peach—look for light-to-medium, clear colors, and avoid all muted, brownish shades. Also avoid blue-pinks or fuchsias, as they are much too cool for you.

If you chose peach as your everyday basic, you'll now need a warm pink or coral pink to wear with your pink clothing. By the same token, if pink is your basic, select a peach or apricot to go with the peach side of your wardrobe. And then add the salmon. You will love having all three of these colors to enjoy with your Spring clothing.

Next, look for a coral in a slightly bright shade to wear with your brighter clothing.

Finally, look for a red. Some Springs, especially brunettes and redheads, wear a clear orange-red beautifully. If you want it a bit less bright, try toning it down by applying pale peach on top. Softer Springs need a lightly frosted poppy shade. If you are afraid of red, you can try a sheer red lip gloss; but most Springs look perkier with a touch of real color, rather than gloss, on their lips.

LIP PENCIL

Make your next purchase a lip pencil, even if you've never tried one. Lip pencils are invaluable, both for giving lips definition and for keeping lipstick from "bleeding" at the edges. They can also be used to cover the lips entirely as a base for lipstick or lip gloss. With a lip pencil foundation, color will stay on all day.

Choose a lip pencil that matches your lipstick color closely so your outlining won't show. If you want to minimize your lips, use a pencil that is slightly deeper than your lipstick. To make your lips look fuller, use a pencil that is lighter than your lipstick. You can also soften the look of a bright lipstick with an outline of lighter pencil; or, if you want a softer lip color, but don't want to look faded, line with a deeper pencil and fill in with the soft color. Always be sure to blend the lipstick over the liner to completely to obscure your outlining. A sharp line looks unnatural and harsh.

You can create "new" shades by covering your lips with pencil and adding various shades of lipstick on top. For example, you might cover your lips with your season's red liner and then apply a cool pink or a warm peach lipstick over it to create an exciting blend. Try it! It's fun to play with your colors.

LIPSTICK TONERS

You might also want to purchase a lipstick toner—yellow gold for Autumns and Springs, silvery white for Summers and Winters. These gleamers are usually slightly frosted and are terrific for toning down bright colors or for creating shimmering new shades. They can also be used right in the center of your lower lip, on top of your lipstick, to give you a "pout."

CHOOSING THE RIGHT FORMULA

Lipsticks come in cream and frosted formulas, usually in tubes, but sometimes in little pans that require a brush for application. Cream lipsticks range from those with lots of pigment, hence thicker coverage and stronger color, to sheer colors that, while not transparent, give a lighter, softer effect. Generally, the thicker creams stay on better because of the extra pigment and thicker wax. The sheers have a moist, shiny look, due to their higher oil content, but they do not stay on long. Some women prefer them for their lighter feeling on the lips as well as their softer color—but you do have to reapply them more often.

Frosted lipsticks have a pearlized, sparkly look and usually provide opaque, rather than sheer, coverage. The pearl content ranges from minimal to extreme. Most women can wear a slightly frosted shade, especially at night, but few but the very young will be flattered by a highly frosted lip color. Frosted lipsticks stay on well, because they are a bit drier, and the color usually doesn't change on your lips after you've worn it a while, the way some creams do.

Lip gloss is sheer and transparent, and comes in a tube, a wand, or a pot. It doesn't stay on long, but gives a subtle, natural hint of color and keeps the lips moist.

Lip pencils are made with much harder wax and less oil than lipstick. Consequently they stay on well, but they can dry your lips if you use them to cover your entire lip area.

If your lips are pale, you will probably prefer the more opaque lipsticks that cover well—the creams or frosts—for their greater color impact. If you have lips that are naturally rosy, or if you prefer subtle lip color, you'll like the sheer lipstick formulas or lip glosses best. Try different formulas to find your favorite. Some companies offer their colors in several formulas to give you a choice.

Lipsticks tend to have three potential problems: "bleeding," breaking, and drying the lips.

- Lipsticks bleed for two reasons—the formula or your lips. The sheer, moist, formulas (especially in red or darker colors) tend to run more easily, especially in hot weather or on a woman with oily skin. If your lips do not have distinct ridges as boundaries, or have feathery lines around the edges, you will have more trouble with lipsticks "bleeding." To correct the problem, choose a harder cream formula, one that pulls a bit as you apply it, or a frost. Or avoid moisturizer around the edge of your mouth, use a lip pencil to outline your lips, and powder your lips before applying the color.

- Lipsticks that consistently break usually have a formula that is too soft. If you love the color, but it gets too squishy every time you buy it, write the manufacturer and tell him. He can adjust the formula, and probably will if he gets enough complaints. Don't leave your lipsticks in a hot car during the summertime. Wax is wax, and it can only take so much heat without melting.

- Lipsticks that are drying or make your lips peel usually have formulas that contain a lot of talc or other fillers to compensate for a lack of pigment. Try changing brands, and avoid frosts, since they tend to be a bit drying. In the wintertime, your lips may dry out no matter what lipstick you use, especially if you have dry skin. Try treating your lips at night with vitamin E, or applying aloe vera gel before you put on your lipstick. (Vitamin E is too greasy to wear under your lipstick. The color will slide right off.)

Now you can see why cosmetics companies guard their formulas so carefully. All women want a lipstick that is moist and creamy but also stays on and doesn't bleed. Contradictory traits! To make a lipstick stay on, it must be made from a harder wax, with less oil, and will necessarily be a bit drier and less shiny. And to have the moist, creamy look, a lipstick will have to sacrifice its staying power. Ah, for the perfect mixture!

INGREDIENTS AND SENSITIVITIES

In addition to oil, wax, and pigments, lipsticks contain fillers, binders, preservatives, and (usually) fragrance to mask their musky smell. Frosted lipsticks also contain mica.

All lip products are not created equal. Some formulas contain extra, protective ingredients, such as PABA (sunscreen), or vitamins A and E (conditioners and emollients).

Natural waxes, such as beeswax and carnauba wax, are especially desirable because they give lipstick a lovely texture and help it smooth on evenly. Price is no guarantee of quality, so you'll have to check the labels to find your favorite ingredients.

If you have an allergic reaction to a lipstick, or your lips burn or swell, look first to the fragrances and preservatives. To identify preservatives, look for words ending in "-paraben." Other additives that can prompt reactions include lanolin, PABA (even though it's good, some people are allergic to it), and coloring agents. If you're having trouble, change to a different color, a different brand, or try a hypoallergenic formula. If you can isolate the offending ingredient, read labels and simply avoid it.

APPLYING LIP COLOR

The first key to beautiful lips is definition. Some women have lips with a natural outline around the edges. Most of us, however, have lips that blend into our faces and really need to be outlined with a lip pencil or a lip brush. Whether the color is soft and subtle or bold and dramatic, it's definition that gives us that elegant, finished look.

It is imperative that you apply your lipstick straight and evenly, especially at the corners of your mouth—another convincing reason to use a lip pencil or a brush to outline your lips! Nothing looks worse than a messy swipe of color that leaves your lips crooked and unbalanced.

Your goal is luscious lips with a natural line and shape. If you feel your lips are too full or too thin, or if the corners turn down, I've included some special tips at the end of this section. Here are the easy steps for applying your lipstick perfectly every time. Use the same principles for lip gloss.

1. With a lip pencil or a lipstick brush turned sideways to make a thin line, draw along your upper lip line from the outer left corner to the center, and then from the outer right corner to the center. If you are more comfortable working from the center to the corners, that's fine, too. But never draw one continuous line from left to right, or your lips will be crooked. Follow your natural lip line and don't make the bow of your lip too pointed. The peak of the bow is usually under your nostrils.

2. Next, draw your lower lip line, again from each corner in to the center.

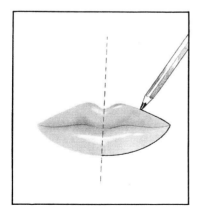

3. Now, fill in with your lipstick or gloss. You can apply either straight from the tube, bringing the color right up to your liner, or you can dab it on with a brush. A brush is handy because it lets you control the coverage, making it as thick or thin as you like. If you've used a lip liner in a different shade from your lipstick, blend it well so its edges don't show.

4. Check to see if your lips look straight. If you've gone over or under the boundaries

here and there, simply touch up and straighten with your lip pencil or brush.

5. To make your lipstick stay on longer, blot your lips, powder them, and then reapply the color. The talc from the powder will help your lipstick cling. Apply gloss on top if you want a shiny finish. (Do not powder your lips if you are applying lip gloss by itself.)

6. Look at your total face in the mirror and see if the colors are in balance—cheeks, eyes, lips. Perhaps now that you've added lipstick you need a bit more blush. If not, your makeup is finished!

Special tips

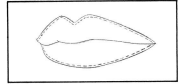

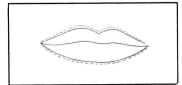

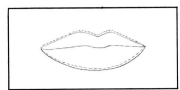

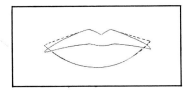

If your lips are full, try applying your lip pencil just *inside* your natural lip line. Remember, you can also use a lip pencil darker than your lipstick to help the narrowing effect.

If your lips are thin, extend your lip pencil just *outside* your natural lip line. A pencil lighter than your lipstick will give your lips a little extra fullness, too.

If your lips are unbalanced, apply the liner just *outside* your natural lip line on the thin lip, just *inside* on the full lip. Refer to the contouring section in Chapter 8 for more tips on balancing lips.

If your lips go downward on the ends, you can give yourself a "lift" by slightly raising the corners of your lips. Here's how. Either pencil in the corners of your upper lip to turn upward, or stop the corner short on the upper lip so the lower lip extends at the corners. Either technique will give the illusion of lips that "smile" at the corners. Don't overdo.

Don't carry any of these strategies too far or your lips will end up looking comical. If people can see that your lips are drawn on, the distraction will counteract any benefits you were hoping for.

Now practice! The effort will quickly pay off. Soon applying lipstick will be second nature, and you'll be able to do it perfectly in one minute or less—small effort for such glamorous results!

Now, with your makeup done, how do you feel? I hope the answer is "Fabulous!" You deserve that wonderful feeling—to hold your head a little higher, to stand a little taller, to straighten your shoulders—just to bask in a warm glow of confidence. Why not feel proud of the way you look, worthy of being noticed and happy to show off the beautiful creation that you are?

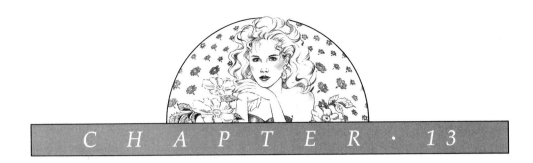

Evening

Evening is your chance to sparkle and to add a little drama to your makeup. Low, flattering lights allow you to deepen or brighten your colors without appearing overdone. Shimmering, frosted shades inappropriate for day wear look subtle and beautiful by candleglow. At night you can let your imagination run to more glamorous effects.

As always, your season will guide you in choosing your colors for nighttime dazzle.

STEPS FOR A BEAUTIFUL EVENING

When the evening is special, allow extra time to take a relaxing bath and to apply your makeup carefully. Plan ahead so you can treat your face to a scrub and mask that will leave it tingling and radiantly clean. After toning as usual, begin your makeup magic:

1. Apply your foundation (a *little* heavier, if you wish) to cover any flaws.

2. Next, cover any circles under your eyes, lines around mouth and nose with concealer. Pat to blend. (At night you may prefer to apply concealer first, under your foundation, for extra coverage.)

3. Contour the hollows under your cheeks by patting on a darker foundation with your contour sponge, or brush on pressed powder in a darker shade, blending the edges. Give your nostrils a bit of flare by brushing darker foundation in the bevels at either side of the tip of your nose. You might want to follow some of the tips in Chapter 8 to sculpt other areas of your face.

4. Now powder your entire face. Dip your powder blush first in your blush, then in your powder, and add a subtle glow of radiance to your whole face.

5. Apply blush as usual. With your fan brush, sweep a brighter shade, for extra glow, right on the crest of your cheekbone.

6. You can line your eyes a little more dramatically than usual. Now's your chance to use black (if your lashes are dark) or a color such as blue, green, or violet to enhance the color of your eyes. Or, use a neutral on the bottom and a color on your upper lashes. (Again, balance the color with your coloring. A woman with blond hair and lashes does not look attractive with heavy black eyeliner, even at night.)

7. Apply your eye shadow as usual, but now you can use frosted shades. Also, try using a deeper color than your daytime shadow, or simply top off your regular shade with a deeper or brighter shade just on the outer corner of your lid. Start with your highlighter and cover the eye area. Add your glamorous color to the outer third of your lid, blending it up onto the outer third of your eyebrow only as far as the end of your brow. Now apply a medium to dark shade across the rest of your orbital bone. This contour shade should not be frosted, especially if your bone protrudes.

8. Now for a note of sparkle: Apply a pale frosted or iridescent "stripe" of shadow to the center of your eyelid, placing it directly over your pupil. Try silver or pearly pink for the cool seasons, gold or frosty peach for the warms. (If

your eyelids show a lot, use a medium neutral shade in a minimum frost instead.) The shimmery shadow will catch the light as you move your eyes, making them magnetizing. Blend the gleaming shadow into the edges of the darker shade.

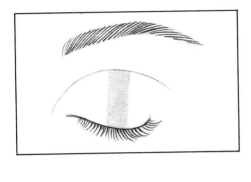

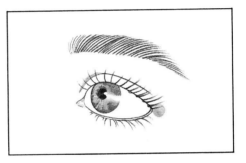

If you have room on your upper brow bone, apply another dot of frost just under the arch, blending it well, to lift the eye.

Add a third glimmer at the outer edge of the eye, right in the crease, just under your darker shadow, to lift your eye. Blend the dot upward to dispel any droopiness.

9. If your eyes are not sensitive, line the rim of your lower lid inside your lashes with a kohl pencil in the same color as your liner. (Be sure to use a pencil that is safe for use near the eye.) Lining the inner rim will make your eyes look slightly smaller, but they will look more dramatic. If your eyes are very small, try lining the inner rim with a white pencil instead, which will make the whites of your eyes look bigger. If you don't feel comfortable putting makeup on your inside rims, feel free to skip this step.

10. Next, apply your mascara—the first coat. Separate your lashes with your brow/lash brush and let the mascara dry.

11. Powder your entire face again, including the eye area, with loose, translucent powder, using downward strokes. You are looking smooth and flawless by now.

12. Now dust on some more luster: Use your fan brush to apply loose iridescent powder—silver for the cool seasons, gold for the warms—and sweep it across your cheekbones, the tips of your nose and chin, and over your upper forehead. With a clean eye sponge, apply the iridescent powder more heavily along the top of your cheekbone (but not into the circular area under your eye).

   If you prefer, you can lightly dust your entire face with iridescent powder. And if you are bare-shouldered, shimmer it across your shoulders and your collarbone, too.

13. Apply your second coat of mascara and separate your lashes with your brow/lash brush. By now they should look full and luxuriant.

14. Finally, it's time for lipstick. You can use deeper or brighter shades than your daytime color, balancing them with the color of your clothing. For example, Winter's black dress calls for red or deep pink lips; while a Spring's pastel ensemble calls for medium to pastel lip color. In the center of your lower lip apply a dab of frosted silver or golden lip gleamer to give yourself a charming pout. For a gleaming, moist finish, cover your lips with clear gloss.

15. Check yourself in the mirror to see that the colors of eyes, cheeks, and lips are in balance. Use powder to tone down an area; add more color to brighten. Perfect.

Feeling glamorous? You are!

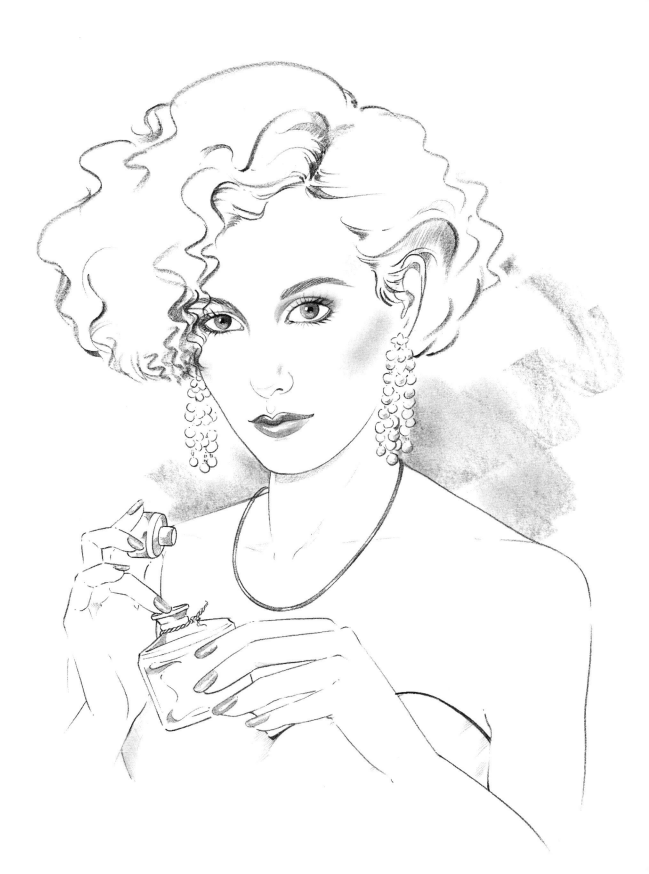

Part III

Finishing Touches

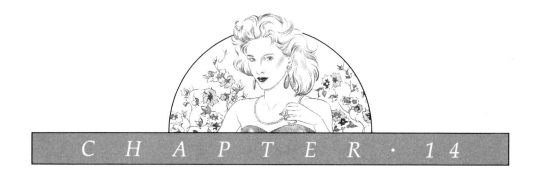

Nails

Many of us let our fingers do the walking and our hands do the talking, yet don't even consider them in our beauty rituals. Next to your face, there is no other part of your body that is so much in the public eye. I have seen women who, at first glance, look impeccably groomed, only to notice later that their nails are chipped and their hands look rough.

None of us wants unattractive hands, but most of us do not want to spend a lot of money on a professional manicure. With a few supplies, some simple guidelines, and less than an hour of time, you can do a perfect manicure at home that will last for a week at least. Isn't that worth it?

CHOOSING THE RIGHT COLORS

Your nail color should match or blend with your lip color, so you can use the lipstick colors from your season's palette as a shopping guide for purchasing nail colors as well. If you plan to wear a variety of colors during the course of any given week, you will need to wear a versatile shade of nail polish—one that will blend with most of your lipsticks and the colors in your wardrobe—and save those bright reds, fuchsias, or corals for special occasions. (Or plan your wardrobe a week at a time so you are wearing all colors that will go with, say, red lipstick and nail polish.) If your nails are short, they will look better in softer, neutral colors rather than dark or bright ones.

Safe shades for each season are:

Winters: a medium rose or strawberry shade, one that blends with both reds and pinks.

Summers: a soft rose or soft strawberry, again to bridge the spectrum between red and pinks.

Autumns: a mocha or tawny peach, fairly muted, so it will go with your soft colors as well as your reds.

Springs: a soft salmon, not too pink, not too orange, to cover the span of your wardrobe.

To assure that your nail polish stays fresh and applies smoothly, you want to take a few precautions. First, keep your bottles of nail color away from heat because heat will thicken the polish—plus, it's highly flammable. You can keep it fresh the longest if you store it in the refrigerator!

Nail color will "bubble" if it is applied too thickly and not allowed to dry between coats, if it is applied in the wind or sun or too close to a heat source, or if it is too old or thick. If you have a bottle of favorite nail color that has thickened, you can buy polish thinner. Don't try to thin your polish with polish remover. The ingredients are totally different, and it won't work.

NAIL-CARE PRODUCTS

To give yourself a manicure that lasts, you'll need to assemble the proper tools and products. If you don't already own them, you'll find these items available in most drugstores. You'll see when to use each as we go through the steps for a perfect manicure.

Polish Remover

Polish remover comes in bottles for use with cotton balls, or in sponge-filled jars into which you dip your fingers and rub the nail against the sponge. I recommend nonacetone formula, as it's less drying to your nails and cuticles.

Cotton Balls

Cotton balls come in two sizes. The larger ones are more practical for polish removal.

Emery Board or Diamond File

Your emery board or nail file is used to shape your nails and maintain their desired length. The emery has a rough and a smooth side, is made of woody fibers and will wear out with use. The metal diamond file lasts longer, but doesn't file your nails as smoothly.

Liquid Cuticle Remover

Cuticle remover is used to soften your cuticles and help "float" off the dead skin.

Cuticle (Orange) Stick

A cuticle stick is pointed at one end and flat at the other. Originally made from orange wood, these are used to push back the cuticle and will not damage the matrix, which is the part from which the nail grows. A damaged matrix can cause the nail to grow out lumpy and irregular.

Base and Top Coats	Base and top coats are both important and each has a specific use. The base coat holds the color on the nail and the top coat seals it from damage and makes it last longer.
Nail Polish	Polish comes in cream and frost formulas. Either is fine, though cream is more appropriate for the office. A good brand should stay on for five to seven days, depending on what you do with your hands. Obviously, scouring pots and pans will shorten the life of your manicure, no matter how good the polish.
Rich Hand Cream	Use a hand cream or body lotion that's extra rich and special for your manicure. You can even use your favorite moisturizing cream.
Cuticle Cream	Cuticle cream is thicker than hand cream. If you rub it on your cuticles every night, it will help preserve your manicure and keep your cuticles smooth and lovely.
Cuticle Clippers	Cuticle clippers are used to clip hangnails or jagged bits of cuticles. They come in both scissor-type handles or palm-grips. Use whichever is more comfortable for you, but shop for as good a pair as you can afford. Used as described below, they prevent many a painful nail disaster.

STEPS TO A PERFECT MANICURE

Now it's time to hide the phone, turn on some music, and make those fingers match the rest of your Color Me Beautiful image!

1. Assemble the tools listed above and, in addition, gather the following items.
   - Bowl of warm, sudsy water
   - Bowl of warm, clear water
   - Two hand towels

   Place one hand towel out flat on your table and arrange the other supplies on top.

2. Remove your old nail color. Dampen a cotton ball with polish remover and remove every last trace of old color. Don't forget the area closest to your cuticles. Even if you aren't wearing nail color, it's a good idea to do this step anyway to remove any traces of oil or cream.

3. Shape your nails with your emery board or nail file. It is important to shape them when they are dry because wet nails are weaker and can be easily damaged. File them from the outside edge in to the center, avoiding a back-and-forth sawing motion, because this can weaken your nails. Be careful not to file into the cuticles at the corners. Your nail shape should follow the contour of the ends of your fingers rather than be too pointed or squared.

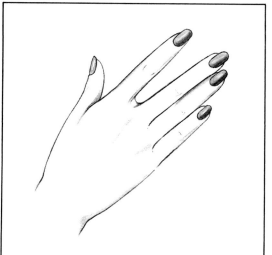

File your nails so the shape follows the contour of your fingertips—oval rather than pointed or square.

4. Soak your nails in the warm, sudsy water for three minutes to soften the cuticles and loosen dirt that may have become imbedded beneath the tips of your nails. Use the pointed end of your cuticle stick to remove dirt. Then blot your hands on your towel.

5. Now apply your cuticle remover according to the directions on the bottle and allow it to remain on for three to five minutes. Using the wedge-shaped end of your cuticle stick, gently push back your cuticles. Then swish your nails in the sudsy water and massage them to remove any residue. Rinse your nails in the warm, clear water, and then *dry them well*, gently using the towel to finish pushing back the cuticles.

6. Before you continue, wrap or "twist" a small amount of cotton around the end of your cuticle stick. You may need to use this later dipped in polish remover to "erase" any nail color that gets onto your cuticles. (Cotton swabs are too fuzzy for this purpose.)

7. If you have any hangnails or a cuticle that is jagged, clip the snag ONLY. Do not cut your cuticles otherwise, or they will become rough and jagged all the time.

8. Apply base coat. This step is important in assuring that your polish will adhere better, go on smoother, and not stain your nails. This one step can make the difference in how long your manicure will last! The base coat will remain slightly tacky, and will have a dull finish. Apply base coat from the base of your nail to the tip using three strokes—one in the center and one on each side. Using a lot of little strokes or reapplying in areas already covered will cause a "lumpy" application and will delay drying time. Allow the base coat to dry for one minute. If your nails have ridges, apply a second coat.

9. Now apply polish using the same three-stroke method. Allow the first coat to dry for three minutes, and then apply a second coat and allow it to dry for five minutes. If any polish gets on your cuticles, now is the time to carefully use your cuticle stick moistened with polish remover to "erase" your mistakes.

10. Apply top coat in the same three-stroke method, "wrapping" it over the tip of your nail to protect the edge of the nail color. Allow your top coat to dry for at least fifteen minutes. This is one case when more is better, so a half hour or more is terrific, if you can spare the time! (You can try one of the new "quick-dry" products to speed up the drying process.) To assure that your manicure lasts as long as possible, *repeat this step every day.* (It will only take the top coat five minutes to dry on a daily basis.)

11. When your nails are thoroughly dry, massage a rich hand cream into your hands. The backs of hands have no oil glands, so concentrate cream there and around your cuticles.

On a nightly basis, apply cuticle cream to each nail. Keep the cream by your bedside so you'll get in the habit of using it. It only takes a few seconds and your cuticles will stay smooth and lovely, which not only looks and feels better, but also lessens the amount of time it takes to do your next manicure!

SPECIAL PROBLEMS

Some of us are born lucky, with nails that grow like weeds and never seem to break. Others have nails that break or split easily and are harder to manage. All of us, from time to time, may have special problems in keeping our nails attractive. Here are the most common problems and their solutions.

Yellowing Nails: Chemicals used in film processing, topically applied medications, and darker nail color dyes can turn nails yellow. Always use gloves when working with chemicals, wash hands well after applying medications, and use a base coat before applying nail polish. You can remove some of the yellow staining by soaking your nails for a few minutes in lemon juice.

Breaking, Peeling, Splitting Nails: These problems can be caused by heredity and also by damage to the cuticle or matrix. Be especially careful not to damage your matrix with the nail clippers when snipping problem spots. Also, overfiling your nails at the corners can cause weakness, so you will need to file your nails slightly more squarish to give the sides added strength. Constant exposure to water, as well as dryness from climate, detergents, or chemicals can cause nails to be brittle. It pays to use gloves when doing harsh chores and to use a good hand cream to moisturize your hands and nails. If they are already abused, try an extra-rich cuticle cream at night or rub a coat of baby oil or petroleum jelly over your hands and cuticles, slip on cotton cosmetic gloves (found in drugstores), and sleep with them on. The warmth of your body combined with the oils will help soften and lubricate your skin, cuticles, and nails.

In addition, you may want to try the special polishes called "nail hardeners," made specifically for problem nails. They are usually sold with special base and top coats as well, and they do seem to help.

And try to remember not to use your nails as screwdrivers, lid openers, or pot scrubbers!

Ridges and "Funny" Colorations: Horizontal ridges may reflect a past illness, especially one with a fever, or damage to the matrix, and will eventually grow out. Vertical ridges are genetic and also tend to occur as we age. Gentle buffing, a liquid ridge filler, and/or two coats of base coat can all help smooth out the surface of your nail.

Variations in color can indicate a health problem. If you are light-skinned, your bare nails should match the back of your hand; if dark-skinned, the palm. Anemia can turn nails white; heart or lung problems can make them look blue. Are your nails half-white, half-pink? This could indicate a kidney ailment. If you notice any unexplained change in your nails, see a doctor for answers.

Nail Biting: This is a hard habit to break since often you are not even aware you are doing it. It really helps to keep your nails and cuticles smooth from any tempting snags or rough edges. I have a friend with a nail-biting teenage daughter who treated her to weekly manicures until her nails had grown out. It worked! Not only did the manicures keep the area smooth, but a further incentive was the immediate gratification of seeing her hands look better.

Applying false nails can also give your nails protection from your teeth, and an immediate improvement in their looks, but there is one caution. As the false nails begin to fall off, they can take a layer of natural nail off with them, leaving your nail weaker than ever. If you decide to wear false nails, be sure you buy the appropriate nail remover to dissolve the glue—and not your nail—when you want to remove them.

It's a great idea if you can set aside a weekly time to manicure your nails, maybe while you watch your favorite TV show. With your cuticles kept in good condition, a manicure will take only half an hour. I know I always feel extra good about myself when my nails and hands look their best.

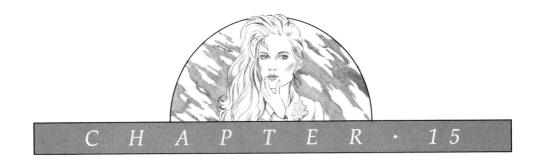

Hair

Whenever I teach a makeup class, invariably I am asked, "What shall I do with my hair?" It's a great question. Most of us don't feel good about ourselves if we don't feel good about our hair. Even with makeup on, we cannot achieve an image we love if we feel our hair is unattractive.

Hair requires two considerations: color and style. Both are important, but for different reasons. Color should flatter and harmonize with our skin and eyes. Style creates balance and line.

COLOR

Nature gives us the hair that goes with our coloring. For many of us, the color we have now is the best. However, many women want to cover gray, stay blond, or simply enhance their natural hair color.

To enhance your hair color, you must choose a color that complements your skin tone. Your natural hair color is your best guideline. Totally changing your hair will detract from the beauty of your skin tone. The wrong hair color will clash just as badly as wearing the wrong makeup colors. Your skin may look muddy, sallow, or even dirty.

Maintaining the blond hair you had as a child or covering gray hair is easy if you use your season and your original hair color as a guideline.

Hair coloring products abound, ranging from color that can be washed out to dyes that change the hair permanently until new hair grows in. Here is a list of the most common types.

Temporary color: Mousses and shampoos have no peroxide, ammonia, or any other chemicals to penetrate the hair's outer layer. They consist of pigment (mixed with water) that stays on the hair surface. They are designed only for subtle changes and for short-term use. They will wash out—or even brush out—quickly. Never use these products immediately after a permanent or other chemical process because the hair has then been made porous and will grab with unnatural intensity.

Semi-permanent color: These have little or no peroxide and simply coat the outer shaft of the hair, primarily with a waxy lotion and pigment. They gradually wear off each time you shampoo. The advantage is that they do not strip the hair and expose red or yellow pigment—especially important for the cool seasons, Winters and Summers, who do not want red tones. The disadvantage is that they do not last as long as permanent color.

Permanent color: These products contain peroxide or other chemicals that penetrate the hair shaft and actually change the hair's natural color. The chemical strips the color from dark to light. Depending on the length of time the product is left on, the hair goes through the following changes in color, starting from black or brown: dark red, orange-red, orange, coin gold, yellow gold, yellow, pale yellow, white.

After the peroxide or stripping agent works, the pigment then penetrates the hair with a new color. Often this is a one-step process, with both the chemical lightener and the pigment deposits doing their jobs at the same time. *Frosting,* however, is a two-step process. First it's necessary to strip the hair of its natural color, to the pale yellow stage. Then the desired shade of blonde is applied. *Streaking and highlighting* are one-step processes. The hair is simply stripped to the desire level of natural pigment and left at that. *Pearlizing* is stripping selected hair in streaks to the white stage, giving a strong contrast most effective for blondes who want a "pearly" blond effect, or Winters who want a shock of white through the bangs.

Some of the permanent products have more peroxide and less pigment, while other brands have more pigment, less peroxide. The brands with more peroxide tend to bring out more red and are best for Autumns and Springs or blond Summers. Cool seasons are best with the low peroxide/high pigment brands.

The advantage of permanent hair color is its longevity. However, in a few weeks the hair oxidizes, and gradually the stripped, reddish hair shows through, a problem for the cool seasons who want to avoid red or gold tones.

With this information, and knowledge of your desired goal, you and your hairdresser should be able to achieve the look you want. On the following pages you'll learn the perfect hair colors for your season. Whether you want to cover gray, stay blond, or simply enhance your natural color, using the right color is the secret to successful results. I have often seen just the tiniest change in hair color improve a woman's looks dramatically!

WINTER

A Winter usually has brown or black hair. She looks wonderful with her dark hair because it provides the contrast that is so becoming to her. She would do best to leave her hair as is. She should never dye her hair blond or red, as these golden tones are unflattering to her skin and her wardrobe. Occasionally, a Winter is born with platinum blond hair that remains blond. It's a striking look, and she needn't alter it. Achieving platinum hair with the bottle is less desirable because it looks artificial and the dark roots show so quickly.

If a Winter craves red hair, she can use an eggplant or violet-based rinse rather than an orange-red tone. The purplish cast, if subtle, will blend with her complexion. Often a Winter can slightly darken her hair to add further contrast and drama. Be careful not to overdo, or the look will be harsh. A vegetable product, such as henna, in a clear or black or eggplant shade can be attractive; it adds shine and depth but maintains the cool highlights she needs.

If your hair turns orange from a permanent, you may need to color it brown again to maintain a cooler shade. If your hair is not damaged, use a semi-permanent product or a low peroxide permanent one.

Winters should avoid frosting or highlighting. Frosting will dull their looks, making them look gray and older. The peroxide used for highlighting or frosting will bring out orange or gold, unharmonious with Winter skin. A black-haired Winter can create a thick, dramatic streak through her bangs by stripping the hair all the way to white (pearlizing). If you can only succeed in achieving blond rather than white, forget it. It won't look good.

To cover gray, a Winter should again avoid red tones. Always look for products that say "ash" rather than "warm." To cover a small amount of gray, use the semi-permanent products with no peroxide. Choose a shade *lighter* than your existing brown hair; otherwise, your brown hair will get darker too, and the overall effect will be too dark. Once your hair is mostly gray, you can use a permanent product, preferably a brand with a high-pigment content. Choose a color as close as possible to your original color. If your hair was black, you will need to settle for dark brown; solid black dye looks harsh on anyone. It's a good idea to leave a little gray showing for softness. The hairdresser can wrap some strands of your gray hair in foil and keep it from being colored.

A Winter will often gray in a silvery tone, a salt-and-pepper look, or pure white. The effect can be so beautiful that you may want to leave it natural.

SUMMER

Summer women, like Winters, want to maintain an ashy tone to their hair and avoid red tones. Even though a few Summer brunettes have red highlights, these highlights will by nature be purplish rather than orange. Like Winter, a Summer brunette would do best to leave her hair natural. The beautiful ashy tone (which she often calls "mousey") looks gorgeous when she wears her palette of cool colors in makeup and wardrobe. If she insists on red tones in her hair, she should use only a subtle eggplant shade, avoiding any hint of orange.

Most Summer women who were blonds through their teens want to stay blond. Blond hair will look great because these Summers have a blond complexion and don't need dark hair for contrast. Be sure to choose an ash or pale beige blond tone but do not overdo and turn your hair ashy green. You can still be a yellow blonde; just avoid the yellow that is brassy or golden. If your hair is light brown, you may want to frost your hair to achieve a blond effect. Have your hairdresser strip your hair to the pale yellow stage, and then apply a soft beige, champagne, or ash blonde to the frosted strands.

Be careful not to become so blond that you lose all the contrast your hair gave you, thus making your face pale. If you are naturally a light blonde, nature will have made your complexion to go with it. But if you are light brunette, your skin needs some contrast, so choose a dark blond shade or leave some brown mixed with the blond to add depth.

Summer women usually gray to a dusty silver, blue gray, or a pearly white shade. A Summer brunette who is graying can simply return her hair to its original brown or a shade slightly lighter. To cover small amounts of gray, use a semi-permanent product in a light brown shade. If your hair is mostly gray, you can use a permanent product to obtain a truer and more lasting color. Like Winter, avoid reddish or warm shades. Look for colors labeled "ash," "beige," "champagne," or "cool." Avoid "flaxen," "honey," "golden," "red," or "warm."

If you were a blonde, you can strip the gray to a pale yellow and apply blond toner. Or try a reverse frost: color some of the gray hair a light brown, leaving the rest. If your hair has turned a pearl white, either leave it as is or cover with a champagne or ash blond toner.

Some Summers gray in a salt-and-pepper fashion, similar to Winters. If you are so lucky, you may want to leave it natural. Nature has given you that expensive frosted look so many women strive to achieve. Other Summers, once completely gray, have a subtle bluish cast to their hair. It, too, is beautiful as is.

AUTUMN

Autumn women are lucky. Because they look great in warm hair colors, they can have fun coloring their hair. Most Autumns, whether blondes, brunettes, or redheads, have either red, copper, or gold highlights in their natural hair color. Because hair coloring products tend to bring out red or gold in the hair shaft, the Autumn doesn't have to worry. Choose products that say "warm," "honey," "gold," "red," or "copper." Avoid ash or cool shades.

Brunette Autumns can either leave their hair its natural color or use vegetable dyes or rinses to bring out red highlights. You can usually even become a full-fledged redhead if you want to. I know of several Autumns with almost black hair who, after they went gray, colored their hair red. It looked even better than their original dark color!

Auburn and redheaded Autumns can deepen their hair color if they want to enhance the red tones, or they can use streaking to bring out red or golden highlights. Some coloring techniques create several layers of different colors, which can be beautiful on these warm-season beauties. Your hairdresser can strip the sections of hair to various stages of copper, red, orange, and gold.

Light golden brown or blond-haired Autumns should choose golden colors. Streaking is great because it leaves some of the dark blond or light golden brown hair for depth and contrast. Streaking is better than frosting on Autumns because it's bolder, with a broader modulation, rather than the overall two-tone effect of frosting. Blond Autumns need richness to avoid looking pale. Have your hair-dresser strip your hair to the yellow or coin gold stage, but not lighter. You want a metallic, golden look.

Autumns' gray is slightly yellowish or an oyster white. If you are a blonde, your gray will look blond too, and you really don't need to cover it. If it looks truly gray, and you feel older or simply don't like it, then return it to a golden blond.

Redheaded and brunette Autumns, in the graying stages, usually look better when they cover the gray. It's easy to cover your gray because you can wear all the warm hair tones so well. Choose a color just a shade lighter than your original color of red or brown. You can leave a gray shock or two in the bangs and at the temples to give an elegant, sophisticated look and keep the frame of your face a bit softer. Once your hair becomes heavily gray, it can be a beautiful, muted, dusty shade, most attractive with all the warm colors in your palette.

If your hair has turned oyster white, it can look wonderfully dramatic. Unless it makes you feel older, leave it. If you want to color it, you may need to go for a light brown rather than blond. The blond may look too soft and Springlike, and you'll lose the impact you had with white. You will have to experiment with shades.

SPRING

Spring, like Autumn, looks terrific in warm hair tones and can easily color her hair with success. She does not, however, want the metallic look of Autumn. What looks rich on an Autumn will look brassy on a Spring. Spring instead strives for soft, warm tones.

Brunette and redheaded Springs look terrific as they are. You can lighten your hair a bit, if you like. Avoid getting too coppery or you will look like an Autumn. Your skin demands delicacy, even if your hair is dark. Vegetable dyes or rinses are good because they just add sheen and a hint of color. Highlighting to lift the color here and there is fine also. A Spring does not want to darken her hair because then she risks looking harsh.

Many Springs were blondes in childhood. A few even stay flaxen blond throughout their lives. Most, however, begin to darken during their teens. If your face needs contrast, it's best to leave your hair darkish and add streaks for the blond effect you like. If you still have a blond complexion, you can certainly go ahead and be a blonde.

To achieve Spring blond, your hairdresser should strip your hair past the coin gold stage to yellow or pale yellow. You can apply colors ranging from beige to clear, light yellow blonde. An overall blonding looks great on Spring, because she looks good in brightness and clarity. Thick streaks of pale blond "sunlight" will also work well, especially if her roots are brown and she doesn't want the hassle of coloring her hair every week or two. Frosting is too muted a look for Spring.

Spring's gray has an ivory cast or even a reddish tinge. Many light-haired Springs actually look blond as they gray because the gray is so yellow. If you are lucky enough to have "blond" gray or to have a head of solid ivory white hair, leave it as is if you're comfortable with it. If you are a dark brunette Spring or a deep redhead, you are better to cover the gray. The two-tone look is not flattering. Once completely gray, your brightness returns.

To cover gray, color it a soft golden blond, red, or light brown, depending on your original hair color. If you are covering only a small percentage of gray, choose a shade lighter than your original color. You don't want the nongray hair to become too dark. Once you are mostly gray, choose a shade closer to your original color, or lighter, as you prefer. Often, brunette Springs look great as blondes once their hair grays.

ALL SEASONS

When coloring your hair, always consider the amount of contrast you need next to your face. Don't make yourself look pale with hair that's too light, or harsh with hair too dark. Soften the shade with age, but dark-haired Winters and Autumns should never go too light—just a shade or two lighter than your pre-gray hair color. You need contrast. All gray hair must be kept relatively short, with a meticulous, stylish cut. Long, scraggly gray hair just doesn't make it. You don't want to look gray and old. You want to look gray and chic.

CHOOSING THE RIGHT STYLE

Your hairstyle says much about you. You tell the world whether you're casual, conservative, sophisticated, or avant-garde by your hairstyle. Sometimes you even tell your age. The woman who still wears a hairstyle that was popular in the 1950s lets everyone know when she went to high school!

It's important to stay up to date, have fun with your hair, and be comfortable. I recommend going to a great hair stylist for an initial cut and styling. You may need to go two or three times to get it just right. Tell the stylist about your life-style, how handy you are with a blow dryer or curlers, and any past experiences you've had with hairstyles. Evaluate what you're working with. Is your hair limp or coarse? Does it frizz in humid weather? Do you have cowlicks that play havoc with a short cut?

Next, tell the stylist what kind of statement you want to make. Use pictures in magazines to illustrate your ideas. Perhaps you're ready to be more sophisticated, or you're just in the mood to try something new. You owe yourself a spiffy style. If you make a mistake, you can always change it! Hair grows. It's fun to have change, and often it takes only a small change to have a great new style. I recall one client who had a permy "bubble" cut—O.K., but a touch matronly. The stylist simply sculpted the hair closer at the nape of the neck, leaving some longish hair down the neck, and presto—an up-to-date look.

*W*rong: Old-style "bubble."   *R*ight: Up-to-date look.

CREATING BALANCE AND LINE

Finally, consider the shape of your face. I find face shape charts to be frustrating and mostly unhelpful. Most faces don't fit them anyway. A rule of thumb is to form your hair to balance the narrow or wide spots and follow the lines of your face.

BALANCE

If your face is narrow, fill in the sides with a fuller hairstyle. If your forehead is extremely high, fill it in with some hair—a few wisps, an off-center part with some hair falling across the side of the forehead, or full-fledged bangs. If your face is extra wide, sculpt some hair across the wide spots and don't have the style too full.

If you have a prominent feature, such as a large nose or a square jaw, flatter the feature rather than try to cover it up. Balance a prominent nose with fullness at the back of the head—a wedge cut, fluffy layers, short full curls, or a chignon, for example. A long, pointed chin looks great with a haircut that is full and rounded, ending at the chin. A double chin is helped by shortish hair that sweeps upward and outward. A small chin is flattered by height at the crown, with the length ending either above or well below the chin line. Flatter a square jaw by exposing it with hair swept back at the temples, and a short cut feathering down the neck, or a longer, angled cut ending below the chin. Don't wear horizontal bangs or have a horizontal cut ending right at the jawline. A square jaw can be balanced by an asymmetrical haircut, exposing the jaw on one side.

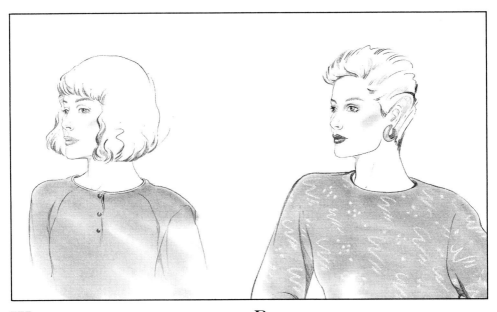

Wrong: Soft, limp hairstyle detracts from angular face

Right: Angular hairstyle complements angular face.

Take the size of your head into consideration, too. If your head is small for your body, have a fuller style. For a large head, choose less fullness.

LINE

The lines of your face give you an automatic direction for your hair. If you have sharp cheekbones and chin, choose a sharp, crisp cut. That's you! The cut can range from severe to slightly curvy, but don't try to change your natural style and "soften" your angles with a limp hairdo. If you have a rounded face, choose a style that has curls or curves, or sweep your hair off your face loosely, rather than tautly. If you have angles, but they're not sharp, you have more flexibility with styles. You can go with either soft, straight lines or curved lines. Very curly hair is best on small to medium-size faces with no sharp features.

Have fun with your features. Don't try to hide them. Go with them rather than against them. Your hair will be not only flattering but also a mark of your self-confidence. Let your hair show off your personality!

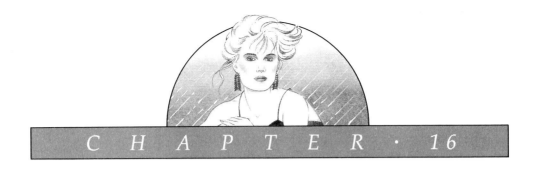

Fragrance

Many women tell me they don't feel completely dressed without fragrance. Indeed, fragrance is the finishing touch in completing the image you have carefully created with your makeup and your wardrobe. Not applying your fragrance is like painting a beautiful picture and neglecting to frame it.

Your season gives you the perfect guidelines for finding that special fragrance that will be your trademark, or for acquiring a wardrobe of fragrances to reflect your every mood. Women of the same season tend to have similar pigmentation and oil content in their skin, and these factors affect how a fragrance will react on you. Haven't you ever noticed that a scent you admired on someone else just didn't work on you?

In addition, fragrance evokes color. Master perfumers, those talented artists who design the perfumes that become our heart's desire, use colors to describe the mood and makeup of their creation. A fresh, outdoorsy scent is green and yellow.

An exotic Oriental fragrance is red and black. Romantic, sweet scents are violet, pink, pastel, and soft white, while rich, sensual fragrances might be fiery red, orange, and gold. Often the colors on the package or perfume bottle denote the mood of the fragrance inside.

I spent two years researching and designing our four Color Me Beautiful fragrances. I grew to love the whole concept of fragrance because it appeals to all our senses. The individual scents that go into a fragrance are called "notes," just as in music. Flavor is represented through the smell of cinnamon, spice, vanilla, and fruity additions. Sight is conjured in our memory through the scents of woods, greenery, and, of course, flowers. Fragrance embodies our total spirit through smell, sound, sight, touch, taste, and, of course, imagination.

In shopping for fragrance, bear in mind that the "notes" take time to evolve. The top note is the scent you smell first, when you apply fragrance to your skin, creating your first impression. Top notes are volatile and tend to fade quickly. Middle notes begin to appear within a few minutes after application, blending with the top notes. The final notes emerge during the "dry down" phase of the fragrance, and these linger several hours after the fragrance has been applied. The final notes are the main body of a fragrance. To properly evaluate a fragrance, you need to wear it at least one hour, so it's full orchestration can appear.

To create the Color Me Beautiful scents, I worked with a different master perfumer for each season's perfume, so the artist would give his full attention and energy to his creation. We had panels of Winters, Autumns, Summers, and Springs, and our Color Me Beautiful consultants tested our fragrances at our conventions and in their studios and boutiques. We refined our scents until they were perfect, capturing the essence of each season's woman. Now I can tell a woman's season with my eyes closed—by her perfume!

Your favorite signature scent will most likely come from your own season's array of fragrances, but try on some of the other fragrances as well and see how they react on you. Sometimes we want a different mood or personality. Although I am a Winter, there are days when I feel like a sassy Spring, a soft romantic Summer, or a warm and fiery Autumn.

WINTER

The Winter woman, with her darker, more dramatic looks and deeper skin tone, wears Oriental scents beautifully. Warmth and mystery best describe the Oriental fragrance family. Orientals are a mélange of rich notes of musk and amber, lush woody notes of sandalwood and patchouli, embellished by sensuous vanilla or exotic fruits.

In designing "Winter," I wanted to create a mysterious impression. This Oriental fragrance begins with intoxicating top notes of mandarin, spearmint, neroli (citrus), and ylang-ylang. Its unusual and refreshing topnotes are joined by midnotes of jasmine and sensuous rose, with the dry down phase revealing the distinctive notes of vanilla, olibanum, and moss. It's light enough for day, sexy enough for evening. I love it.

In addition to the Color Me Beautiful fragrance, "Winter," other favorite winter fragrances are:

Amber Mist, by Avon	Magie Noire, by Lancôme
Anne Klein II, by Parlux	Oscar de la Renta, by Oscar de la Renta
Aromatics Elixir, by Clinique	Obsession, by Calvin Klein
Ciara, by Ultima II	Paloma, by Paloma Piccaso
Fendi, by Fendi	Shalimar, by Guerlain
Gloria Vanderbilt, by Warner	

SUMMER

The soft, romantic femininity of the Summer woman is best represented by flowery, aldehydic scents. Aldehydes, which create the illusion of pure oxygen (ozone), add sparkle and volume to flowery notes. The ozone effect is not unlike the wonderful aroma that permeates the air in a mountain forest. Beautifully interpreted in 1921 by Chanel No. 5, the flowery aldehydic family is the foundation of many creations, all of which radiate elegance and femininity.

The "Summer" fragrance by Color Me Beautiful starts with a delicate bouquet of narcissus and aldehyde, soon surrounded by intimate and sensual florals of rose, jonquil, and marigold, crescendoing into the magical notes of heliotrope, amber, and a touch of vanilla, which adds a powdery note throughout. Summer, to me, describes beauty through and through.

In addition to the Color Me Beautiful fragrance, "Summer," other favorite summer perfumes are:

Anaïs Anaïs, by Cacharel

Chanel No. 5, by Chanel

Chanel No. 19, by Chanel

Cristalle, by Chanel

Enjolie, by Charles of the Ritz

Glorious, by Warner

Joy, by Patou

Le Jardin, by Max Factor

Liz Claiborne,
  by Liz Claiborne Cosmetics

Lutèce, by Houbigant

Ombre Rose,
  by Jean Charles Brousseau

Private Collection, by Estée Lauder

Rive Gauche, by Yves Saint Laurent

Silences, by Jacomo

AUTUMN

A fragrance that marries the delicate florals and rich semi-Oriental families perfectly portrays the Autumn woman, with her combination of warm femininity and tactile sensuality. Semi-Oriental perfume often presents spicy, woody, and musky notes, the family of scents that is sophisticated and opulent.

For "Autumn" we created a luxurious combination of rare florals. The notes begin with iris and ylang-ylang, enhanced by midnotes of muguet, tagette, and sage clary. Exotic notes of sandalwood, vetiver bourbon, and rich moss complete this magnificent fragrance. It's spicy, woody, and sensual—so Autumn.

In addition to the Color Me Beautiful fragrance, "Autumn," other favorite autumn fragrances include:

Coco, by Chanel

Cabochard, by Grès

Cachet, by Prince Matchabelli

Gucci III, by Gucci

Halston, by Halston

K L, by Karl Lagerfeld

Opium, by Yves Saint Laurent

Poison, by Dior

Ruffles, by Oscar de la Renta

Teatro Alla Scala, by Krizia

Youth Dew, by Estée Lauder

SPRING

The Spring woman is delicate but sensuous, and intensely feminine. She is perfect in a flowery composition that blends different floral scents, subtly combined with green, fruity, spicy, or woody notes. Her fair skin demands a scent that is not too heavy, but her fragrance must nonetheless have presence.

For "Spring" I wanted to create a tender, yet passionate fragrance. Its first impression is of jasmine and honey, leading into essences of hyacinth, honeysuckle, and lily-of-the-valley, laced by warm, sensuous notes of musk, vetiver, and soft amber. Does that sound like you, Spring?

In addition to the Color Me Beautiful fragrance, "Spring," other favorite Spring perfumes are:

Aliage, by Estée Lauder

Beautiful, by Estée Lauder

Anne Klein, by Parlux

Charlie, by Revlon

Colors, by Benetton

Fidji, by Guy La Roche

Giorgio, by Giorgio

L'Air Du Temps, by Nina Ricci

Lauren, by Ralph Lauren

Norell, by Revlon

Paris, by Yves Saint Laurent

Privilege, by Privilege

White Linen, by Estée Lauder

Wind Song, by Prince Matchabelli

Ysatis, by Givenchy

CHOOSING THE RIGHT FORMULA

Fragrance comes in different concentrations. The more oil and less alcohol, the richer and longer-lasting the scent. *Perfume* has the highest concentration of oil and is by far the most expensive. Next comes *eau de parfum* with a fairly high proportion of oil, *eau de toilette*, and then *cologne*, with the least amount of oil and the most alcohol. A woman with dry skin will not have good luck with her scent lasting if she is only using cologne, because neither her skin nor the fragrance has much oil to help the scent linger. She is better off wearing eau de parfum or perfume if she wants her fragrance to stay on all day—or evening.

Fragrance is also available in other forms. Whichever scent you choose, there is more to applying it than simply spraying it on. Here are steps to applying a fragrance so you will be surrounded, but not smothered, by it all day.

Step 1: Bath Products
Bath products come in many forms: shower and bath gel or mousse, milk bath, bubble bath, and either a bar or cream soap. They all very gently cleanse and/or soften your skin while lightly scenting it.

Step 2: After-bath Products
Scented creams, lotions, and powders are great for after the bath. These pamper your body while lightly scenting it. Apply one of the moisturizing products first, then lightly dust with scented powder between and under the breasts, under the arms, and anywhere moisture may collect.

Step 3: Light Fragrance Application
Eau de toilette or parfum or cologne spray is next. To properly apply these, you should still be unclothed. Spray your fragrance above and slightly in front of you, and walk through the "cloud" of fragrance. Spraying it behind you next, simply back into the fragrance. Your body will be lightly dusted with fragrance, but not overpowered by it.

Step 4: Perfume
By now, you are very lightly scented from head to toe with your chosen fragrance. Now for the crowning touch, the real thing! Nothing else smells quite like perfume. Dab a tiny bit on several of your pulse points—in the soft spots

just behind your earlobes, on either side of your throat, on the back of your neck, between your breasts, inside your wrists, in the crooks of your arms, behind your knees, and on the insides of your ankles.

Step 5: Refreshing Your Scent

Perhaps at midday, and certainly again before you go out in the evening, you will want to refresh your scent. Dabbing more perfume on your pulse points will bring your fragrance alive again. Keep a bottle or jar of scented lotion in your desk drawer, and massage some well into your hands just before you go out the door. You never know who is going to kiss your hand!

FRAGRANCE DON'TS

As lovely as fragrance is, there are a few "don'ts" to remember.
- Do not spray directly onto your clothing. The oils and alcohol will damage your garment, and the scent never smells as lovely on clothing as on you.
- Do not apply a fragrance on bare skin before sunbathing. It can cause pigment discoloration of the skin.
- Do not wear too much. You want people to notice you first, not your perfume.
- Wear a lighter concentration of your fragrance, or a lighter fragrance, during the summer. Heat intensifies a fragrance.
- Store your perfume in a reasonably cool environment.
- Don't apply perfume with the stopper of your perfume bottle. You risk bringing oils and bacteria from your skin back into the bottle.

ALLERGIES

I can hear some of you: "I love fragrance, but it makes me sneeze. How can I wear it?" First, use perfume instead of lighter concentrations, as it has no propellant and less alcohol, both of which can cause sneezing (and even headaches). Apply it to the back of your neck, shoulders, and knees only, so it won't always be right under your nose. If you still have a problem, try a different scent. You may be allergic to one of the synthetic or natural oils present in one fragrance but not another. If you have a problem with allergies to perfume, sometimes just skipping it during allergy season when pollen counts are high will help.

Wearing fragrance is extremely personal, because the same scent will never smell exactly the same on two people. You may want to be known for your signature fragrance or you may want variety, with different scents for different moods or occasions. Whatever your choice, your personal fragrance statement will assure you of creating positive memories of you wherever you go.

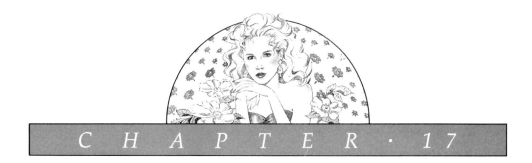

Color Me Beautiful
Inside, Where It Counts

Knowing we look wonderful on the outside has the positive effect of making us feel beautiful on the inside as well. Wearing our colors, makeup, and an up-to-date hairstyle can produce a minimiracle in increased self-esteem.

I'm sure you have seen a transformation in either yourself or a friend who has "found her colors." With her newfound self-confidence, she radiates good feelings about herself. Perhaps she has made major life changes as a result: she changed careers, got a promotion, got married or unmarried, or took action toward accomplishing a goal. At the very least, she is simply happier, and that happiness spreads to everyone around her.

I believe that inner beauty comes from making the most of our God-given gifts. By becoming our best and using our talents we achieve peace and satisfaction.

With increased confidence in ourselves, we often uncover some of our hidden talents because we try things we were afraid to try before.

Whenever I give a speech on personal "success" or using our gifts, invariably several women come up to me afterward to tell me of goals they have buried. One woman gave her "testimonial" to the whole audience. She said she'd always wanted to take singing lessons. She was waiting until her children grew up—but twenty years is a long time to wait. She told us that once she began to feel "beautiful," she started thinking more of herself in other ways, and decided to start singing now. She had just sung a solo in her community theater group and was radiant with self-esteem. Everyone clapped vigorously when she finished her story. We can all identify with buried fantasies!

I hope you will use the tools you have learned in this book to look beautiful on the outside, feel wonderful on the inside, and become truly excited about yourself and your personal gifts. The physical and spiritual parts of ourselves taken together make such a beautiful whole person. Let your outer beauty brighten your life and your inner beauty radiate to all those around you.

Your Beauty
Regimen

The following charts are designed so you can cut them out of the book, staple the pages together at the top, and make a "flip" chart to use as a step-by-step guide as you put on your makeup.

Feel free to place the Concealer Chart ahead of the Foundation Chart, if you prefer that order.

Happy makeup!

Love,

Carole

BEAUTY TOOLS

1. Under-eye brush

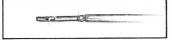

2. Powder brush

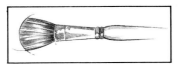

3. Blush brush

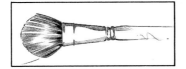

4. Contour brush

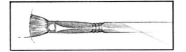

5. Fan brush

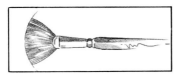

6. Eyeliner brushes

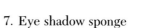

7. Eye shadow sponge

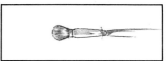

8. Eye shadow brush

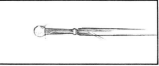

9. Eye contour brush

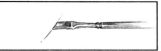

10. Brow and lash brush

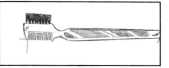

11. Lipstick brush

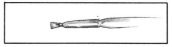

SKIN CARE

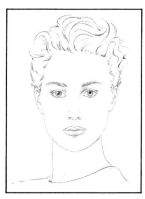

SKIN-CARE REGIMEN

	Dry	Normal/Combination	Oily
Step 1	Eye makeup remover Cleanser—cream or liquid • Gentle scrub • Honey mask, once/week	Eye makeup remover Cleanser—liquid or facial soap • Scrub, once/week • Mud mask or honey mask, as needed	Eye makeup remover Cleanser—facial soap • Scrub, twice/week • Mud mask, once/week
Step 2	Toner	Toner/astringent	Astringent
Step 3	Cellular renewal or other nourisher	Cellular renewal or other nourisher	Cellular renewal or other nourisher
Step 4	Rich moisturizer or night cream	Light moisturizer or night cream if needed (Repeat toner)	Moisturizer on neck only or where needed (Repeat toner)
Step 5	Eye cream	Eye cream	Eye cream

FOUNDATION

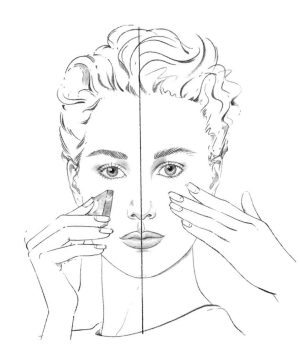

WATER OR OIL BASE

Dot on makeup using corner of sponge. Blend with sponge, using downward and outward strokes. Be sure to cover eye, lip and area around nose. Blend carefully at jawline.

OIL FREE

Stipple on and feather with fingers to blend, using downward and outward strokes. Avoid eye area. Let dry. "Buff" with a dry cosmetic sponge. Apply oil-base foundation to eye and lip areas.

EYE SHADOW BASE: You can apply eye shadow base instead of foundation to brow and lid area. Dot and blend.

TIP: Color adjuster: Before applying foundation, feather green color adjuster over ruddy areas, lavender adjuster over sallow cheeks, forehead, chin. Let dry. Follow with foundation.

CONCEALER

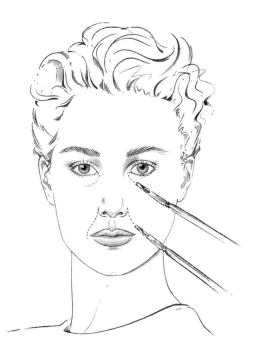

MINIMAL PROBLEM: Using under-eye brush, apply coverstick sparingly on top of foundation. Feather on dark areas *only*. Pat with fingertip to blend.

SEVERE PROBLEM: *Before* applying foundation apply concealer to dark areas. Then apply foundation, patting gently so concealer is not removed.

FACE SCULPTING

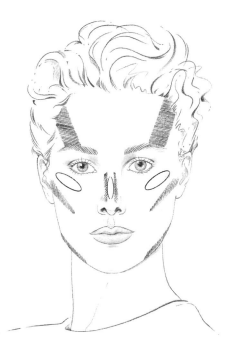

- Apply highlighter down center of nose and at crest of cheekbones.

- Apply contour shading to sides of nose, bevels at tip of nose, hollows of cheeks and to forehead above outer half of brow.

- If your upper lip is thin, apply a thin rim of highlighter along edge of lip.

- Blend so effect is subtle. (Face sculpting is best for evening.)

POWDER

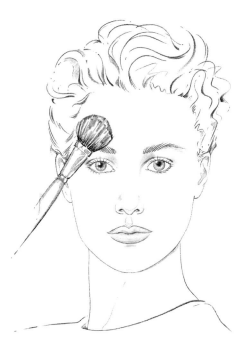

1. Sprinkle powder in palm of hand.

2. Dip brush in powder and shake off excess.

3. Brush on forehead first, then cheeks, nose, chin, and eyes, using downward strokes.

TIP: To add overall glow, dip powder brush lightly in blush, then in powder. Brush over entire face.

BLUSH

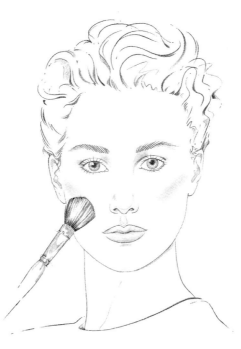

1. Apply blush along cheekbone, starting right under outer edge of iris, feathering into hairline at top half of ear. Do not cover top of cheekbone or go below hollow of cheek.

2. Blend edges with contour brush.

NARROW FACE

Apply blusher from outer edge of eye, blending back (not up) toward center of ear.

WIDE FACE

To slim face, bring blush slightly farther forward and lightly lower, with sharper upward angle toward top of ear.

EYELINER

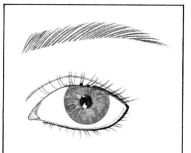

LITTLE OR NO LID SHOWING

Line entire lower lid and outer third of upper lid. Use this technique if no lid shows whether your brow is large or small. Blend to soften.

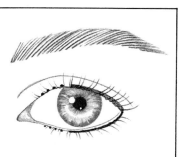

PROPORTIONED: LID AND BROW ARE APPROXIMATELY EQUAL

Line outer half of upper and lower lids, feathering edges toward nose so the line doesn't end abruptly. Blend liner to soften.

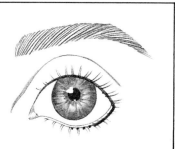

PROMINENT LID, SMALL BROW AREA

Line entire upper lid and outer third of lower lid, feathering lower edge so it doesn't end abruptly.

Blend and "smudge" edges with a clean eye sponge or under-eye brush.

EYE SHADOW

1. HIGHLIGHTER: With your eye sponge, apply a highlighter to entire area, from lashes to brow.

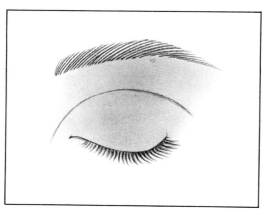

2. SHADOW COLOR: OUTER LID: Using your eye contour brush, apply contour shade to outer third of lid.

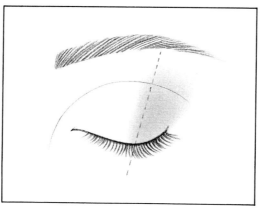

3. SHADOW COLOR: ORBITAL BONE

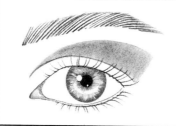

1. *Proportioned: Lid and brow area approximately equal.*
Apply contour shadow above the crease, from outer eye to inner, concentrating most of the color on the outer two thirds of the orbital bone. Blend toward the brow. Apply a pale uplifter color to the inner two thirds of your lid. Blend. If your lid shows a lot, use a soft neutral, not a lighter bright color.

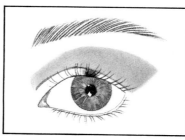

2. *Little or no lid showing; more brow area.*
Apply contour shadow to orbital bone in a half-circular shape, raising shadow higher toward brow in the center. Blend upward and outward toward brow. Place a dot of uplifter on lid just above iris. Blend slightly.

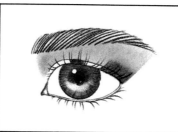

3. *Little or no lid showing; small brow area.*
Apply a pale color on the entire area from your crease to your brow. Sweep a little of the darker shadow from the outer corner of your lid up toward the end of your eyebrow. Dot uplifter on lid.

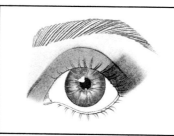

4. *Prominent lid; small brow area.*
Apply a light shadow on bone above crease, blending it up toward brow. Apply a medium neutral shadow on inner two thirds of lid. Blend. Now brush a little of the darker eye shadow from the outer corner of your lid up toward the end of your eyebrow.

TIP: If eye shadow seems too dark, blend entire area with contour brush, stroking upward; dust with translucent powder.

/

MASCARA

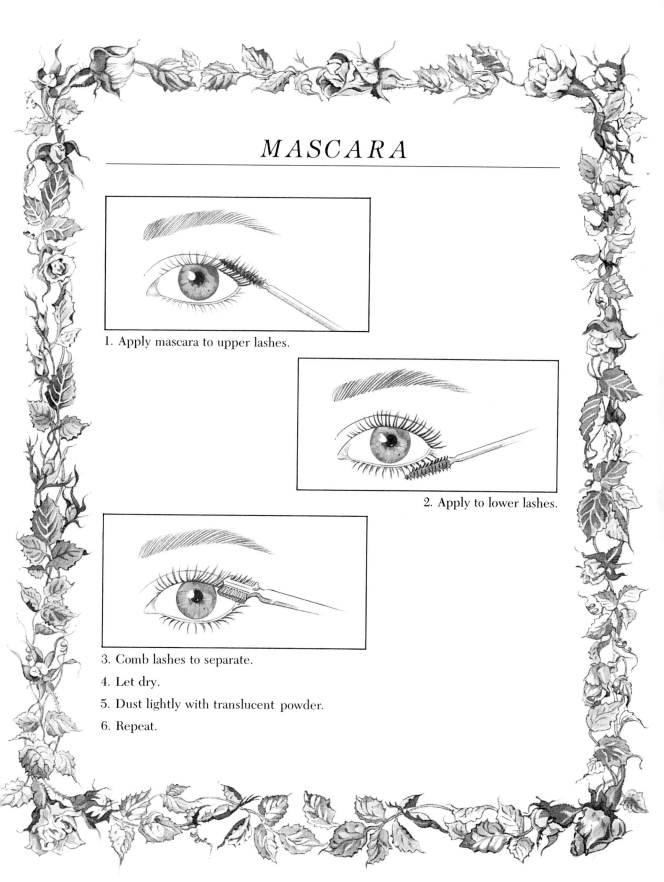

1. Apply mascara to upper lashes.

2. Apply to lower lashes.

3. Comb lashes to separate.

4. Let dry.

5. Dust lightly with translucent powder.

6. Repeat.

EYEBROWS

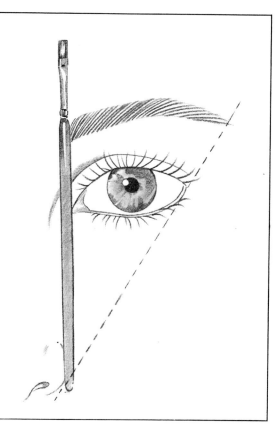

1. SHAPE:

With your brow/lash brush, brush brows upward and then smooth outward.

2. BROW DEFINER

Using the same boundaries you use for plucking your brows, feather in pencil or brow powder to fill in length or bare spots.

LIPSTICK

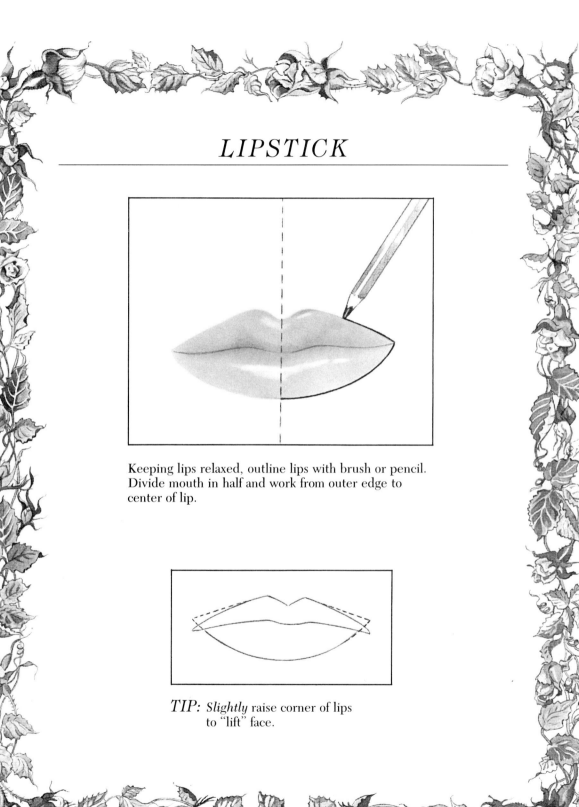

Keeping lips relaxed, outline lips with brush or pencil. Divide mouth in half and work from outer edge to center of lip.

TIP: *Slightly* raise corner of lips to "lift" face.

YOUR FINISHED LOOK

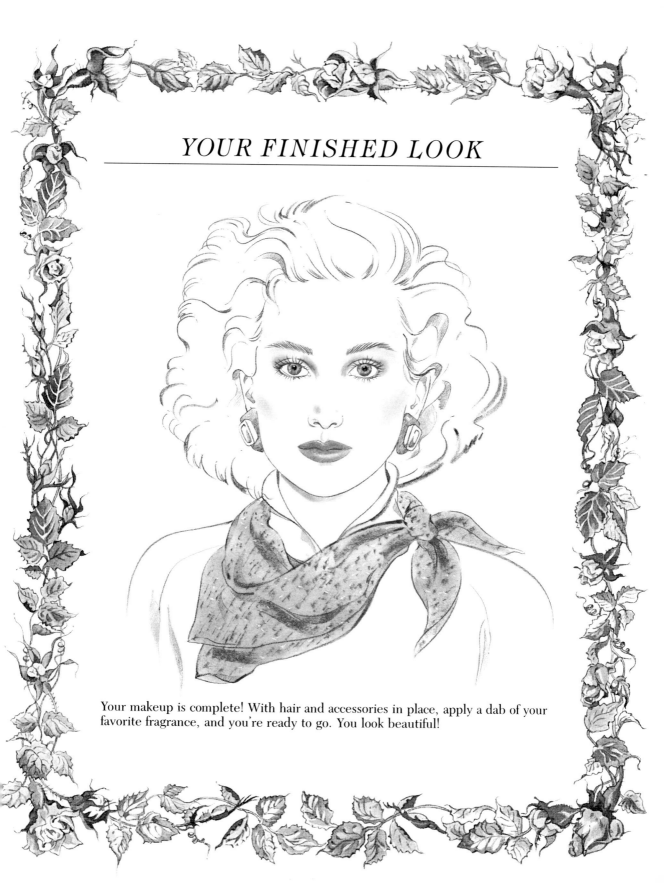

Your makeup is complete! With hair and accessories in place, apply a dab of your favorite fragrance, and you're ready to go. You look beautiful!

EVENING

1.
Freshen nose with foundation.

2.
Contour hollow of cheek.

3.
Powder entire face. For a subtle overall glow,
dip your powder brush first in your
blush, then in your powder.

4.
Perk up blush with brighter color on cheekbone, if desired.

5.
Use iridescent powder over cheekbone, if desired.

6.
Freshen eyelid with frosted shadow.

7.
Freshen orbital bone with deeper color.

8.
Touch up lashes with mascara on tips, if needed.

9.
Refresh lipstick. Add gleamer to center of lower lip.

WINTER MAKEUP WARDROBE CHART

Clothing Color	Lipstick	Blush	Eye Shadows	
			Highlighter	Contour Colors
All Pinks Magenta Royal Purple Icy Violet				
True Red Blue Red				
Fuchsia				
Bright Burgundy Vivid Cranberry				
Lemon Yellow Icy Yellow				
Bright Periwinkle Blue Royal Blue True Blue Icy Blue				
Hot Turquoise Chinese Blue Clear Teal Bright Emerald Turquoise Icy Aqua				
Light True Green True Green Emerald Green Pine Green Icy Green				
Black White Navy All Grays				
Black-Brown Taupe				

SUMMER MAKEUP WARDROBE CHART

| Clothing Color | Lipstick | Blush | Eye Shadows | |
			Highlighter	Contour Colors
All Pinks All Roses Lavender Orchid Medium Violet				
Watermelon Red Blue-Red				
Soft Fuchsia				
Plum All Mauves Raspberry Burgundy/ Maroon				
Light Lemon Yellow				
Powder Blue Sky Blue Cadet Blue Medium Blue Periwinkle Blue				
All Aquas Soft Teal				
All Blue Greens Spruce Green				
Grayed Navy Grayed Blue Light Blue-Gray Charcoal Blue- Gray				
Soft White Rose Beige Rose Brown Cocoa				

AUTUMN MAKEUP WARDROBE CHART

Clothing Color	Lipstick	Blush	Eye Shadows Highlighter	Contour Colors
Orange-Red/Bittersweet Dark Tomato Red				
Brown Burgundy Mahogany				
All Peaches/Apricots				
Orange/Pumpkin Terra Cotta Rust				
Light Gold/Buff Gold Golden Yellow Mustard				
Purple Aubergine/Eggplant				
Salmon Pink Salmon				
Teal Blue Turquoise Jade Green				
All Periwinkle Blues				
Bright Yellow-Green Forest Green Olive Green Moss Green Grayed Green				
Oyster White Warm Beige Khaki/Tan Camel Coffee Brown Dark Brown/Charcoal Medium Warm Bronze Warm Gray/Pewter				
Marine Navy				

SPRING MAKEUP WARDROBE CHART

| Clothing Color | Lipstick | Blush | Eye Shadows | |
			Highlighter	Contour Colors
Warm Pastel Pink Coral Pink Clear Bright Warm Pink Medium Violet				
Clear Salmon				
Bright Coral				
All Peaches/Apricots Light Orange				
Orange-Red Clear Bright Red				
Buff Light Clear Gold Bright Golden Yellow				
All Yellow-Greens Light True Green Kelly Green				
All Periwinkle Blues Light True Blue Medium Blue				
All Aquas Emerald Turquoise Light Teal Blue				
Ivory Light Warm Beige Camel/Tan Medium Golden Brown Chocolate Brown				
Light Warm Gray Medium Warm Gray Light Clear Navy Clear Bright Navy				

Index

BEAUTY ON THE GO MAKEUP KIT

Now that you know your season, you may want to have our purse-size makeup kit in your season's colors! Each kit contains two lipsticks, two blushes, and four eye shadows in colors for your season, plus applicators. Your kit comes in a colorful "lizard skin" cover: purple for Winters, pink for Summers, turquoise for Autumns, and yellow for Springs.

FABRIC SWATCHES
FOR YOUR CLOTHING WARDROBE

To help you coordinate your wardrobe with your makeup colors, you may want a set of thirty-six fabric swatches, in the same color lizard skin wallet as your makeup kit.

FINDING OR BECOMING AN IMAGE CONSULTANT

If you need help determining your season, you can get the names of the Color Me Beautiful consultants nearest you. If you would like to become a consultant yourself, there are opportunities available for qualified applicants.

For information on any of the above, write or call:

Carole Jackson
P.O. Box 3241
Falls Church, VA 22043
(703) 560-7111